# Young Children
# With ADHD

# Young Children With ADHD

## EARLY IDENTIFICATION AND INTERVENTION

◆———————————◆

## George J. DuPaul and Lee Kern

AMERICAN PSYCHOLOGICAL ASSOCIATION

WASHINGTON, DC

Published by
American Psychological Association
750 First Street, NE
Washington, DC 20002
www.apa.org

To order
APA Order Department
P.O. Box 92984
Washington, DC 20090-2984
Tel: (800) 374-2721; Direct: (202) 336-5510
Fax: (202) 336-5502; TDD/TTY: (202) 336-6123
Online: www.apa.org/pubs/books
E-mail: order@apa.org

In the U.K., Europe, Africa, and the Middle East, copies may be ordered from
American Psychological Association
3 Henrietta Street
Covent Garden, London
WC2E 8LU England

Typeset in Goudy by Circle Graphics, Inc., Columbia, MD

Printer: Maple-Vail Books, York, PA
Cover Designer: Berg Design, Albany, NY

The opinions and statements published are the responsibility of the authors, and such opinions and statements do not necessarily represent the policies of the American Psychological Association.

Library of Congress Cataloging-in-Publication Data

DuPaul, George J.
 Young children with ADHD : early identification and intervention / George J. DuPaul and Lee Kern. — 1st ed.
    p. cm.
 Includes bibliographical references and index.
 ISBN-13: 978-1-4338-0963-7
 ISBN-10: 1-4338-0963-X
 1. Attention-deficit hyperactivity disorder—Diagnosis. 2. Attention-deficit hyperactivity disorder—Treatment. 3. Attention-deficit-disordered children. I. Kern, Lee. II. Title.

 RJ506.H9D85 2011
 618.92'8589—dc22

                                    2010042151

British Library Cataloguing-in-Publication Data

A CIP record is available from the British Library.

Printed in the United States of America
First Edition

doi: 10.1037/12311-000

# CONTENTS

# PREFACE

Attention-deficit/hyperactivity disorder (ADHD) is a disruptive behavior disorder that involves the display of developmentally inappropriate levels of inattention, hyperactivity–impulsivity, or a combination of these characteristics (American Psychiatric Association, 2000). Children with ADHD typically experience significant difficulties with social behavior and academic achievement that increase the risks for conduct disorder, delinquency, and poor educational outcomes (Barkley, 2006). It is a disorder of relatively high prevalence (5%–10% of the child population) and requires long-term treatment with behavioral strategies and possibly medication. Until recently, most research regarding the assessment and treatment of ADHD has focused on elementary school–age children, despite the fact that ADHD symptoms and the associated impairment often begin early in life. As a result, young children with ADHD frequently enter school at a significant behavioral and academic disadvantage relative to typically developing peers. Thus, since the start of the 21st century, there has been increased attention to the difficulties, needs, and treatment of preschool-age children (i.e., 2–5 years old) with or at risk for ADHD.

Together with our colleagues and students at Lehigh University and Lehigh Valley Health Network, we have developed and investigated a comprehensive early intervention program for young children with ADHD. The primary goal of this program is to prevent, delay, or reduce the negative functional outcomes typically associated with early ADHD, such as conduct problems (i.e., aggression and rule-breaking behavior), difficulties with early reading and math skill development, and problems interacting with peers and adult authority figures. In particular, we tried to address the cross-situational nature of ADHD by implementing behavioral and academic intervention strategies across home and preschool settings. Thus, the early intervention program involves parents and teachers working together over an extended time period (i.e., a year or more) to provide a consistent approach to addressing ADHD and related difficulties.

In the course of our research, it became clear that not all children required the complete early intervention protocol. Some children improved sufficiently once their parents implemented behavioral strategies under our direction. Others required the full intensity of treatment across settings for an extended period of time. Thus, we designed a three-tiered approach to early intervention that is based on models used in special education and school psychology (e.g., schoolwide positive behavior support; Horner, Sugai, Todd, & Lewis-Palmer, 2006). The objective of the multitiered approach is to focus appropriate levels of treatment resources according to children's needs (i.e., to individualize treatment). The level or intensity of treatment necessary for each child is individually determined on the basis of his or her response to intervention at each tier. The components of this multitiered approach, as well as challenges with implementation, are discussed in detail in this book.

We provide here a detailed description of our early intervention for ADHD program as well as the outcome data that we have collected thus far in support of this model. The volume addresses a clear need in the ADHD literature because we know of no other book specifically devoted to early intervention with this population. The book is intended for mental health and education professionals who work with young children with challenging behaviors, especially ADHD, including school psychologists, clinical child psychologists, special educators, social workers, and counselors. It may also be useful in graduate courses in early intervention or related topics. Although our efforts to develop a successful, cost-effective early intervention program continue, our hope is that this book will help professionals to design and implement efficacious strategies with families and preschool personnel working with young children with ADHD.

The research underlying the development of the early intervention program described in this book was supported, in part, by several grants from foundation, state, and federal sources. Specifically, we acknowledge support from the D. R. Pool Healthcare Trust, as well as from a Commonwealth of Pennsylvania Tobacco Settlement grant to Lehigh University. Major funding for our research was provided by National Institute of Mental Health Grant R01-MH61563. The opinions and positions stated in this book are those of the authors, and no endorsement by any external funding agencies should be inferred.

We also greatly appreciate the efforts of the many research scientists and assistants who worked on our early intervention research projects, including Kate Ackley, Lauren Arbolino, Charles Barrett, Genery Booster, Amy Boyajian, Rachel Brandt-Greenfeld, Lindsey Brookes, Megan Brotz, Lauren Dullum, Tulani Freeman, Marcie Handler, Jocelyn Helwig, Clarissa Henry, Shelley Hosterman, Suzanne Irvine, Karen Jensen, Anju Kaduvettoor, Anastasia Kokina, Jaana Lehtinen, Rebecca Masters, Kristen Mehr, Karen Neifer, Nina Nonnemacher, Sean O'Dell, Mary Pipan, Katherine Reilly, Catherine Riley, Christy Rothermel, Laura Rutherford, Peter Slay, Natalie Sokol, Lisa Thomas, Brigid Vilardo, and Dongyuan Yu. We are especially grateful to our primary collaborators on these research projects, including Grace Caskie, J. Gary Lutz, John Van Brakle, and Rob Volpe. Kristen Carson provided critical assistance with literature searches and tracking down relevant research.

Finally, we are grateful to the many children, parents, teachers, and health care professionals who participated in our early intervention research projects. Needless to say, their efforts were critical to the successful development of a comprehensive early intervention protocol. Thus, we dedicate this book to the participating children and families in the hope that future generations of young children with ADHD can benefit from early intervention.

# Young Children
# With ADHD

# INTRODUCTION

The symptomatic behaviors of attention-deficit/hyperactivity disorder (ADHD) significantly compromise the behavioral, family, academic, and medical functioning of young children. The difficulties associated with ADHD typically begin at an early age and are usually unremitting (Lahey et al., 2004; Massetti et al., 2008; Pierce et al., 1999). Diagnostic advances allow for increased accuracy in early identification, and thus, the best opportunity to prevent significant deficits, reduce the need for medical intervention, and boost academic readiness skills involves intervention during early childhood. Findings from our prior National Institute of Mental Health (NIMH)–supported study, coupled with additional emerging research, provide preliminary evidence of substantial improvements with early childhood intervention. There is a strong theoretical and empirical rationale for identifying young children with or at risk for this disorder to reduce concurrent difficulties and prevent more serious negative outcomes.

ADHD is a disruptive behavior disorder characterized by developmentally inappropriate levels of inattention and hyperactivity–impulsivity (American Psychiatric Association, 2000). Boys with ADHD outnumber girls with this disorder, ranging from a 2:1 ratio in school-based epidemiological studies to 5:1 or higher among clinic-referred children (Barkley, 2006). ADHD is associated with significant academic, social, and occupational impairment that is evident throughout the life span for most affected individuals (Barkley, 2006). As a result, the development and implementation of effective interventions are of paramount importance, with a recent impetus to identify and treat the disorder as early as possible.

The purpose of this Introduction is to provide an overview of ADHD, particularly as it relates to the functioning of young children (i.e., ages 2–5 years). First, the *Diagnostic and Statistical Manual of Mental Disorders* (4th ed., text revision; *DSM–IV–TR*; American Psychiatric Association, 2000) criteria for ADHD are described in terms of how symptoms may be manifested in young children. Second, areas of impairment associated with ADHD in early childhood are reviewed, including problems with parent–child and family interactions, development of antisocial behavior, deficits in preacademic functioning, and disruptions in the development of peer relationships and social functioning, as well as increased risk for injury and medical care involvement. Next, the typical developmental trajectory for young children with ADHD through childhood and adolescence is described, with particular emphasis on academic, behavioral, social, and occupational outcomes. Fourth, theory and research related to the development of ADHD are briefly reviewed as a rationale for early intervention. Finally, we provide an overview of the content of the remainder of the book.

## ADHD IN EARLY CHILDHOOD

The *DSM–IV–TR* criteria for ADHD include a list of 18 behavioral symptoms that are divided into two clusters. One cluster contains nine inattention symptoms:

- often fails to give close attention to details,
- often does not follow through on instructions and fails to finish work,
- often has difficulty organizing tasks and activities,
- often avoids tasks that require sustained mental effort,
- often loses things necessary for tasks or activities,
- often forgetful in daily activities,
- often does not seem to listen when spoken to directly,
- often easily distracted by extraneous stimuli, and
- often has difficulty sustaining attention in tasks or play activities.

The other cluster includes nine hyperactivity–impulsivity symptoms:

- often fidgets with hands or feet or squirms in seat,
- often leaves seat in classroom,

- often runs about or climbs excessively,
- often has difficulty playing quietly,
- often is "on the go" or acts as if "driven by a motor,"
- often talks excessively,
- often blurts out answers before questions are completed,
- often has difficulty awaiting turn, and
- often interrupts or intrudes on others.

These criteria further stipulate that (a) some ADHD symptoms must cause impairment before age 7 years; (b) some impairment from the symptoms must be present in two or more settings (e.g., home, school); (c) there must be clear evidence of clinically significant impairment in academic or social functioning; and (d) the apparent ADHD symptoms must not be better accounted for by other emotional or behavior disorders, such as autism, depression, anxiety disorder, or schizophrenia. There are three subtypes of ADHD:

- *predominantly inattentive type* (i.e., significant problems with inattention only),
- *predominantly hyperactive–impulsive type* (i.e., significant problems with hyperactivity–impulsivity only), and
- *combined type* (i.e., significant problems with both inattention and hyperactivity–impulsivity).

On the basis of these diagnostic criteria, by definition, children with ADHD must manifest impairing symptoms during early childhood (i.e., before 7 years old). Although issues such as rapid developmental changes between the ages of 2 and 6 years make diagnosis of preschool-age children somewhat tenuous (Lahey et al., 1998), recent research provides evidence that symptoms of ADHD emerge at a very young age (Egger, Kondo, & Angold, 2006; Spira & Fischel, 2005; Sterba, Egger, & Angold, 2007; Wolraich, 2006). For example, in a comprehensive literature review of published research with children ages 2 to 5 years, Egger et al. (2006) found that ADHD symptoms, consistent with *DSM–IV–TR* criteria, can be reliably assessed and occur outside of the normative range for preschool-age children. Further, the ADHD-related characteristics seen in younger children mirror those in older children with respect to prevalence, subtypes, and gender differences, offering added support for an accurate nosology.

Estimates of the prevalence of ADHD among school-age children range from 3% to 5%; consequently, it is one of the most common psychiatric disorders. In preschool-age children (i.e., 3–5 years old), prevalence estimates vary greatly. Lavigne et al. (1996) found a prevalence rate of approximately 2%, whereas Keenan et al. (1997) found that 5.7% of 5-year-olds in a low-income sample met diagnostic criteria for ADHD. In a more recent epidemiological study of disorders in a large, community-based sample of 4-year-olds,

Lavigne, LeBailly, Hopkins, Gouze, and Binns (2009) found ADHD in 6.8% to 15.1%, depending on the severity of associated impairment. ADHD in young children is associated with clinically significant impairment in behavioral, social, and preacademic functioning, with affected children approximately 2 standard deviations below their non-ADHD counterparts in all three areas (DuPaul et al., 2001). In a longitudinal study, Lahey and colleagues (1998) found that preschool children diagnosed with ADHD continued to show functional impairment 3 years later and that symptom severity was the most significant marker of persistence into middle childhood. Together, this research strongly supports the early emergence of a constellation of symptoms characteristic of ADHD that is atypical of preschool-age children, relatively common in this age group, and associated with significant impairment across settings.

Given that ADHD tends to be chronic, at least 70% to 80% of preschool-age children with this disorder will continue to exhibit significant ADHD symptoms during elementary school (Lahey et al., 2004). Children exhibiting high levels of hyperactive and impulsive behaviors (i.e., combined or predominantly hyperactive–impulsive types of ADHD) are at higher than average risk for developing other disruptive behavior disorders (i.e., oppositional defiant disorder [ODD] and conduct disorder [CD]) along with academic and social deficits (Campbell & Ewing, 1990). In addition, 59% to 67% of children with ADHD whose difficulties are persistent at school entry will continue to show significant symptoms of disruptive behavior disorder during middle childhood and early adolescence (Pierce, Ewing, & Campbell, 1999), and nearly 90% will fall short of being considered well-adjusted as adolescents (Lee et al., 2008). Significant ADHD symptoms are associated with chronic behavioral and academic impairment for a large percentage of affected youth. For example, children (N = 303) from the Preschool ADHD Treatment Study (PATS; Greenhill et al., 2006) were found to have significant impairment that was correlated with ADHD severity, with younger children exhibiting the greatest levels of symptom severity. Overall, the majority of the PATS sample (69.6%) had one or more comorbid disorders with ODD, communication disorders, and anxiety disorders being the most common. These data clearly underscore the importance of early intervention to reduce the impact of ADHD and to interrupt the typical sequelae of this disorder.

## CASE DESCRIPTIONS

Four brief case descriptions are provided to illustrate the variety of ways that ADHD can manifest in early childhood, as well as the extent to which functioning in several areas can be affected. These descriptions represent children who were referred to and participated in our early intervention research project (Kern et al., 2007), described later in this text. Here and throughout, identifying characteristics have been altered to guarantee anonymity.

Bobby M. is a 4-year-old, White, non-Hispanic boy who was referred for treatment by his preschool teacher because of his frequent inattentive and disruptive behavior during both structured (e.g., circle time) and unstructured (e.g., free play) activities. He attends preschool 3 days per week for 3-hour sessions. His parents are separated, and he lives with his mother, grandmother, and younger sister. Parent and teacher ratings of his behavior on the Conners Rating Scales—Revised (CRS–R; Conners, 1997) indicate that levels of inattention, impulsivity, and high activity are more frequent than 95% of other boys his age. Further, a diagnostic interview with his mother indicated his behavior meets *DSM–IV–TR* criteria for ADHD—combined type. Although Bobby's teacher reports some noncompliant behavior in the classroom, his behavior does not meet diagnostic criteria for ODD. His score on the Differential Ability Scales (DAS; Elliott, 1990) places him in the low average range of cognitive ability. His scores on the Bracken School Readiness Composite (SRC; Bracken, 1998) and the Social Skills Rating System (SSRS; Gresham & Elliott, 1990) indicate that he is behind his age-mates in academic skills and social behavior, respectively. Specifically, Bobby has experienced difficulties learning and retaining letter-naming and number-naming skills. Further, he has only one friend in his class, another boy who displays similar disruptive behaviors. Bobby's mother reports that his behavior is difficult to control at home, particularly when he is asked to follow rules or complete a task or when he is playing with his younger sister.

Jerilyn S. is a 5-year-old, White, non-Hispanic girl who was referred by her kindergarten teacher. Jerilyn attends a half-day kindergarten program 5 days per week. She lives with her parents and two older brothers. At school, she is reported to have significant difficulty staying seated, maintaining attention to assigned tasks or instructional activities, and getting along with her classmates. At times, Jerilyn is verbally aggressive with her peers and also is openly defiant with her teacher. Parent and teacher ratings on the CRS–R (Conners, 1997) indicate that her inattentive, hyperactive–impulsive, and defiant behaviors are more frequent than those seen in 98% of other girls her age. Further, her parents report symptomatic behaviors consistent with ADHD—combined type and ODD. Although her cognitive ability (as measured by the DAS) is in the average range, she is experiencing some difficulties with early reading skills (e.g., phonological awareness). Teacher and parent ratings of her social skills are in the below average range. Her teacher is concerned that Jerilyn is not making adequate behavioral and academic progress and has suggested that she may need to be retained in kindergarten for the next school year.

Carlos R. is a 4-year-old, White, Hispanic boy who was referred by his mother because of his high activity level and disobedience to parental commands. Carlos lives with his parents, older brother, and maternal grandparents. He attends a half-day prekindergarten program 5 days per week. His preschool teachers describe him as a highly active, curious child who can do well academically when focused. Behavior ratings on the CRS–R (Conners, 1997) indicate that symptomatic behaviors associated with ADHD and ODD occur at a frequency higher than 98% of other boys his age. Parental responses to a diagnostic interview indicate that Carlos's behavior meets *DSM–IV–TR* criteria for ADHD—combined type and ODD. Consistent with the prekindergarten teacher report, scores on the DAS and SRC indicate that he is in the average range with respect to cognitive abilities and preacademic skills. Conversely, teacher and parent ratings on the SSRS are in the below-average range, reflecting significant impairment in his social relationships with peers and adults. His parents report that over the past year, the severity and frequency of Carlos's temper tantrums and disobedience have escalated. In fact, he had been removed from two prior preschool programs because of his high activity level and tantruming behavior.

Scott C. is a 3-year-old boy of mixed racial background who was referred by his outpatient pediatrician because of parental concerns about his high activity level and impulsive behavior at home. Scott lives with his mother and sister and attends a private nursery school 3 days per week. His mother and nursery school teacher report that Scott has difficulty remaining "in one place," frequently interrupts conversations and activities, and is a "daredevil." Parent and teacher ratings on the CRS–R (Conners, 1997) place Scott in the upper 5% of activity level and impulsivity relative to other boys his age. Yet, ratings of attention problems are in the average range. Maternal responses to the diagnostic interview are consistent with a diagnosis of ADHD—predominantly hyperactive–impulsive type and ODD. He is reported to exhibit more than six behavioral symptoms of hyperactivity–impulsivity but only two symptoms of inattention. Scott was functioning in the high average range of cognitive abilities on the DAS and exhibited average-range preacademic skills on the SRC. Alternatively, his SSRS ratings from his mother and teacher were significantly below average, indicating serious difficulties getting along with others and making friends with children his age. His mother and teacher are both concerned with Scott's escalating defiance to commands and physically aggressive behavior with peers, particularly when they are not doing what he wants them to do. He had been removed from two prior preschool programs because of his aggressive behavior and high activity level.

These four case descriptions illustrate several important points regarding the manifestation of ADHD in young children. First, even at a young age, behaviors associated with this disorder affect child functioning in a variety of settings—most prominently, the home and preschool. Second, symptomatic behaviors are evident across the ethnic, gender, and socioeconomic spectrum and are not isolated to any subgroup of the population (although boys are more likely to have the disorder than girls). Third, the disorder is manifested in a variety of forms (i.e., subtypes) and may or may not be associated with other disorders. For example, Carlos's behavior is characteristic of the hyperactive–impulsive subtype because he is reported to exhibit very high levels of physical activity and impulsive behavior, although he does not show significant problems with attention and task engagement. Alternatively, Jerilyn exhibits the full constellation of behaviors comprised by ADHD, and these symptoms meet criteria for the combined subtype. The most common associated disorder is ODD; in fact, 75% of the children in our early intervention research sample exhibited behaviors consistent with both ADHD and ODD. Fourth, inattentive, hyperactive–impulsive, and combined inattentive–hyperactive and impulsive behaviors are associated with significant impairment in academic or social skills (or both). The nature and degree of impairment vary across children; however, it is clear that this disorder places young children at high risk for significant difficulties as they approach school entry. Finally, the attention difficulties, high activity level, and impulsive behavior exhibited by young children with ADHD may lead to removal from preschool or day care programs, further compromising their social and academic skill development.

## FUNCTIONAL IMPAIRMENTS ASSOCIATED WITH ADHD

ADHD symptoms typically persist over time and rarely occur in isolation. As noted earlier, children with the disorder have been found to be more likely than their typical counterparts to exhibit defiant or aggressive behavior across home and school settings, to attain lower than expected levels of academic performance and achievement, and to develop poor peer relationships (Barkley, 2006). Furthermore, young children with ADHD are more likely to sustain physical injuries and receive psychotropic medication relative to their typically developing peers (Lahey et al., 2004).

### Development of Antisocial Behavior

Social development is dependent, at least in part, on the interaction between children's behavioral dispositions (e.g., behaviors symptomatic of ADHD) and parents' behavior management skills (Tremblay et al., 1992). Mothers of young children with ADHD issue significantly more commands, criticism, and punishment than do mothers of non-ADHD children (Barkley, 1988; DuPaul et al., 2001). In addition, mothers of preschool-age children with

ADHD report greater levels of parenting stress than do mothers of similar-age, typical children or even parents of older children with ADHD (DuPaul et al., 2001; Fischer, 1990).

The family is the primary unit of social organization and, as such, has a major influence on children's early cognitive and social development (Levenstein, 1992). The greatest numbers of reinforcers are delivered by those who have the most contact with children (i.e., parents); therefore, positive exchanges with primary caregivers make a significant contribution to children's social development (Patterson, Reid, & Dishion, 1992). A key tenet of Patterson's theory of the development of antisocial behavior (Patterson et al., 1992) is that it begins in the home during the toddler–preschool years. Specifically, children learn that aversive behavior (e.g., crying, defiance) turns off the aversive behavior of parents (e.g., commands). Over repeated trials, children learn to use aversive behaviors as a method to control unpleasant and chaotic situations (Dishion et al., 1992). As children develop, these coercive exchanges intensify in frequency and severity, persist over time, generalize across settings, and result in rejection by parents and peers (J. B. Reid & Eddy, 1997).

Boys with ADHD are 5 to 17 times more likely to develop CD before age 16 than are boys without ADHD (Loeber, Green, Keenan, & Lahey, 1995; Offord, Boyle, & Racine, 1991). Moreover, ADHD is one of the strongest predictors for the early onset (before age 10) of CD (Lahey & Loeber, 1997). Even in epidemiological (as opposed to clinical) samples, there is ample evidence for the central role of concentration problems in setting the stage for aggressive behavior and academic underachievement (Kellam & Rebok, 1992). This is alarming because children with ADHD and early-onset CD typically experience persistent symptoms of both disorders, as well as severe social and academic impairment, throughout their lifetimes (e.g., Lahey & Loeber, 1997; Rutter, 1997).

Although ADHD co-occurs with CD, the association between the two is largely accounted for by accompanying ODD symptoms, at least in males, whereas for females, both ADHD and ODD symptoms contribute to development of CD (van Lier et al., 2007). Consequently, ODD is a key link between ADHD and CD, particularly for males. Furthermore, the risk for CD is greater in children whose parents are not involved in their child's school experience and who are exposed to minimal cognitive stimulation (Hawkins, Catalano, & Miller, 1992).

Therefore, there is a need to enhance parental involvement in the child's academic development and to increase attention to the development of cognitive and preacademic skills. Because parents also are responsible for early cognitive and preacademic skill development, interventions to prevent later school failure must include enhancement of cognitive stimulation by parents (Hart & Risley, 1995; Levenstein, 1992).

Children with ADHD exhibit high levels of disruptive, noncompliant, and sometimes physically aggressive behaviors in preschool or child-care settings (Campbell, Endman, & Bernfield, 1977; DuPaul et al., 2001). These behaviors not only affect interactions with adult caregivers but also may have a negative impact on peer relationships. In fact, peer rejection is strongly associated with aggression, as rated by peers and teachers, among preschool-age children (Milich, Landau, Kilby, & Whitten, 1982). This is not surprising given that children with ADHD who are also aggressive disrupt the play activities of other children and are excessively demanding and noisy during peer interactions (Campbell, Endman, & Bernfield, 1977; Campbell, Schleifer, & Weiss, 1978).

## Development of Literacy and Numeracy Skills

Numerous studies have indicated that children's early experiences with literacy and numeracy have a significant influence on later academic skills. For example, research has demonstrated that children's experience with early literacy activities, such as those that increase phonemic awareness (Snow, Burns, & Griffin, 1998), and early numeracy activities (Gersten, Jordan, & Flojo, 2005) makes a significant difference in their later language and literacy skills and mathematics achievement.

Children entering school vary widely in their phonological awareness and familiarity with and understanding of the alphabetic nature of our language system (Torgesen et al., 1999). Phonemic awareness (i.e., insight that words are composed of sounds) and the alphabetic principle (i.e., ability to associate sounds with letters) are essential for reading acquisition (Wagner & Torgesen, 1987), and children's early knowledge in these areas is highly predictive of later literacy achievement (Foorman & Torgesen, 2001; Torgesen, 2000; Torgesen et al., 2001). Likewise, given the diversity in children's oral language histories and exposure to literature, children enter school with disparate vocabularies (Biemiller, 2001; Hart & Risley, 1995; Snow, Burns, & Griffin, 1998). Vocabulary development is also essential for proficient reading (A. E. Cunningham & Stanovich, 1998; National Reading Panel, 2000; Storch & Whitehurst, 2002).

In addition to literacy skills, early mathematics skills (i.e., fluidity and flexibility with numbers, a sense of what numbers mean, and the ability to make comparisons) are important (Gersten & Chard, 1999). Although findings are still emerging, the preliminary literature suggests that early experience with quantity and numbers may assist children in acquiring critical mathematical skills (e.g., addition, subtraction) once they enter kindergarten (Griffin, 2004).

Several studies have demonstrated that young children with or at risk for ADHD experience difficulties with early literacy and numeracy skills. For example, DuPaul et al. (2001) found that preschoolers meeting diagnostic criteria for ADHD obtained significantly lower scores on a test of cognitive, developmental, and academic functioning compared with a sample of typically developing peers. On average, children with ADHD received scores 1 standard deviation below the expected mean for their age and relative to mean scores obtained by typically developing control participants. This academic achievement gap is similar to that found for older children and adolescents with ADHD (Frazier, Youngstrom, Glutting, & Watkins, 2007) and suggests that academic impairment precedes school entry for many young children with ADHD. Not surprisingly, 3- and 4-year-old children with ADHD are significantly more likely to receive special education services compared with their non-ADHD peers (Marks et al., 2009). In fact, Marks et al. (2009) found that approximately 25% of their sample of children with ADHD received special education services compared with about 5% of children in the control sample.

**Medical Issues**

Young children with ADHD may be more likely to use medical services relative to their nondisabled counterparts for at least two reasons. First, they appear to be at greater than average risk for physical injuries and accidental poisonings, presumably because of high rates of impulsive and overactive behavior (Hartsough & Lambert, 1985; Lahey et al., 1998; Mitchell, Aman, Turbott, & Manku, 1987; Szatmari, Offord, & Boyle, 1989). In fact, Lahey et al. (2004) found that young children with ADHD were 7 times more likely to sustain an accidental injury than their non-ADHD peers when assessed over a 4-year period. Further, the injuries of children with ADHD are more likely to be severe (including loss of consciousness) compared with the injuries of children without ADHD (DiScala, Lescohier, Barthel, & Li, 1998; Lahey, 2000). The relationship between ADHD and accidental injuries appears to be strongest for children with the hyperactive–impulsive subtype (Lahey et al., 1998) and is exacerbated by aggressiveness (Bijur, Golding, Haslum, & Kurzon, 1988; Davidson, Hughes, & O'Connor, 1988). Second, as is the case for older children with ADHD, some preschool-age children with ADHD receive psychotropic medication (e.g., methylphenidate) to reduce symptoms of the disorder. Although exact usage data are not available, Zito et al. (2000) reported a 1.7- to 3.1-fold increase in methylphenidate use in the 2- to 4-year-old age group through the 1990s. Further, 17% of Lahey et al.'s (2004) sample of 4- to 7-year-olds with ADHD were prescribed stimulants in their first assessment wave, with the percentage growing to 48.4% three years later. Thus, it can be assumed that a significant percentage of young children with ADHD are prescribed stimulant medication requiring medical oversight.

For most affected individuals, ADHD is a chronic disorder with symptoms and associated impairment extending across the life span (Barkley, Murphy, & Fischer, 2008). Not only do symptoms persist into elementary school and beyond, but sequelae include academic underachievement, antisocial behavior, risk for physical injury, and long-term receipt of psychotropic medication (see Figure 1).

Preschoolers rated as significantly hyperactive show symptoms that persist into elementary school (Campbell et al., 1986; McGee et al., 1991). For example, Lahey et al. (2004) followed two samples of 4- to 7-year-old children across 4 years, including 96 children who met ADHD criteria and 130 children without ADHD. Cumulatively, 79.2% of children with ADHD continued to meet diagnostic criteria for this disorder at least twice when assessed 2, 3, and 4 years later compared with only 3.1% of the comparison group. The ADHD group also exhibited significantly greater global, academic, and social impairment during Waves 2 through 4 than did non-ADHD control participants. As a result, children in the ADHD group were 3 times more likely to be placed in special education than were their non-ADHD peers, even after accounting for comorbid psychopathology and IQ. ADHD symptom differences (relative to comparison peers) continued to be large over an 8-year assessment period and also predicted significant rates of CD, depression, and anxiety disorder symptoms (Lahey et al., 2007). Finally, young children with ADHD were significantly less likely to be considered well-adjusted in terms of disruptive behavior, peer relationships, and academic achievement when followed into adolescence (Lee et al., 2008). In fact, only 12% to 14% of ADHD probands were considered well-adjusted in adolescence compared with 64.3% to 67.5% of participants in the control group. Thus, ADHD in early childhood is highly likely to persist over time and to be associated with significant functional impairment through elementary school and into adolescence.

Upon school entry, young children with ADHD are likely to be behind their nondisabled peers in basic math concepts, prereading skills, and fine motor abilities (DuPaul et al., 2001; Lahey et al., 1998; Mariani & Barkley, 1997; Shelton et al., 1998). These educational deficits are particularly concerning given the strong relationship between early academic skills and later achievement (e.g., Ferriero & Teberosky, 1982; Kame'enui, 1993). For example, Massetti et al. (2008) followed a sample of 125 children with ADHD, ages 4 to 6 years, across 8 years. Outcome data indicated that they were more likely to show reading, math, and spelling and writing deficits compared with 130 control participants. More specifically, when controlling for IQ, children with the inattentive subtype scored below expectations for all three areas, whereas those with the combined type scored lower than expected for math.

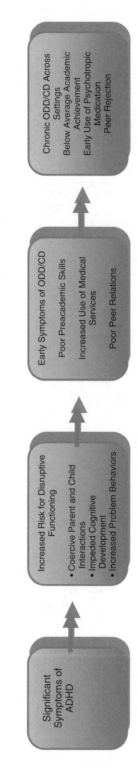

Preschool

Early Elementary School

Significant Symptoms of ADHD

Increased Risk for Disruptive Functioning
• Coercive Parent and Child Interactions
• Impeded Cognitive Development
• Increased Problem Behaviors

Early Symptoms of ODD/CD
Poor Preacademic Skills
Increased Use of Medical Services
Poor Peer Relations

Chronic ODD/CD Across Settings
Below Average Academic Achievement
Early Use of Psychotropic Medication
Peer Rejection

*Figure 1.* Typical trajectory for young children with attention-deficit/hyperactivity disorder (ADHD). CD = conduct disorder; ODD = oppositional defiant disorder.

The meta-analytic findings obtained by Frazier et al. (2007) indicate a mean deficit of .71 standard deviation units between students with and without ADHD, with the relationship between ADHD and academic underachievement persisting into college. The presence of academic (and other) risk factors in children with ADHD is supported by data indicating that young children with ADHD may be at higher than average risk for placement in special education programs during elementary school (Lahey et al., 1998, 2004) and that students with ADHD are less likely to complete high school than their nondisabled counterparts (e.g., Barkley, Murphy, & Fischer, 2008).

Given the ubiquitous and chronic difficulties associated with ADHD, this disorder is costly in terms of lost productivity as well as the use of education and mental health resources. During the preschool years, young children with ADHD receive 2 to 4 times the services (e.g., special education, speech therapy, occupational therapy) of preschool children without ADHD (Marks et al., 2009). Further, Pelham, Foster, and Robb (2007) estimated the annual cost of this disorder to range between $12,005 and $17,458 (in 2005 dollars) per household, with an annual societal cost between $36 billion and $52.4 billion. It is sobering to note that these estimated costs are relatively conservative because some factors (e.g., impact of potential substance abuse, costs associated with adult ADHD) were not factored into the analyses. Clearly, ADHD is a chronic, costly disorder that requires long-term intervention across home and school settings. The difficulties encountered early in life by young children with or at risk for ADHD require early intensive treatment. Emerging research suggests that early intervention could reduce the severity of impairment and minimize costs associated with the disorder over the long term (Kern et al., 2007).

## DEVELOPMENT OF ADHD: THEORETICAL AND EMPIRICAL UNDERPINNINGS

Although it is beyond the scope of this book to review the empirical and theoretical literature regarding the etiology and development of ADHD, it is important to consider evidence that the disorder results from brain and cognitive functioning differences that may be largely genetically based (Nigg, 2006). In fact, the results of family aggregation, adoption, and twin studies indicate that approximately 80% of the variance in measures of ADHD-related behaviors is accounted for by heritable factors (i.e., genetics; Barkley, 2006). The remainder of the variance is accounted for primarily by nonshared environmental factors (e.g., experiences unique to each child). Molecular genetic studies have identified variants of several candidate genes (e.g., dopamine transporter gene, or *DAT1*) as possibly accounting for ADHD symptoms at least in small percentages of the population (Nigg, 2006). Behavioral geneticists postulate that ADHD is most likely related to multiple genes and is not "caused" by a single gene. Most of the candidate genes studied thus far appear to affect the activity of dopamine, a neurotransmitter active in many parts of the brain.

Individuals with ADHD appear to show subtle differences in brain structure and function relative to typically developing peers (Nigg, 2006). Most prominently, these differences are evident in the frontal lobes of the brain, which are believed to control planning and organizational activities. It is interesting to note that the parts of the brain where differences have been found are regions where dopamine is most active, thus tying neurological and genetic findings. It appears, then, that the symptomatic behaviors of ADHD may be caused in part by heritable differences in brain functioning, particularly in parts of the brain that affect impulse control and sustained attention. At the same time, the severity of ADHD symptoms is moderated to a large degree by environmental events and situational factors (Barkley, 2006). For example, children with ADHD do not show high levels of disruptive, inattentive, and impulsive behavior when provided with frequent, immediate feedback. Therefore, the expression of this disorder represents an interaction between inherited brain differences and environmental factors.

The crucial role that the interaction of within-child, biological factors and environmental events plays in determining the severity of ADHD symptoms has led to several theoretical conceptualizations of the deficits underlying this disorder. Despite the primacy of *attention deficit* in the name of the disorder, most theorists do not hypothesize attention as a central, underlying concept (e.g., Rapport et al., 2008). For example, Barkley (1997, 2006) has theorized that the central feature of ADHD is impairment in delayed responding (i.e., behavioral inhibition) rather than a deficit in attention per se. Many important settings (e.g., classroom) and abilities (e.g., internalization of speech) require the capacity to delay responding to the environment. Thus, deficits in delayed responding lead to the exhibition of ADHD symptoms in multiple settings and deleteriously affect the development of rule-governed behavior.

Barkley's (1997, 2006) theoretical model of ADHD as a disorder of behavioral inhibition postulates that impaired delayed responding to the environment compromises the development of four critical executive functions: working memory, self-regulation of affect–motivation–arousal, internalization of speech, and reconstitution (e.g., analysis and synthesis of possible behavioral actions). These executive function impairments in turn lead to myriad problems in cognitive, academic, and social functioning. This theoretical model is supported to a large degree by the extant literature on this disorder (for a review, see Barkley, 2006). This theory implies that interventions for ADHD might include changes in within-child variables (e.g., temporary change in brain functioning through stimulant medication) and/or changes in antecedent and consequent stimuli to increase the probability of delayed responding, thereby leading to attentive, productive behavior (Barkley, 2006). Unfortunately, most homes and preschool settings are structured in a manner that provides delayed, infrequent reinforcement, which are precisely the conditions most likely to lead to inattentive, disruptive behaviors (i.e., impaired response inhibition) in children with ADHD. Thus, the challenge for early intervention is to incorporate environmental stimuli known to enhance child success into settings where impulsive, inattentive behaviors are exhibited.

The preponderance of theory and empirical evidence indicates that ADHD is a disorder that involves an interaction between heritable and environmental factors, is manifested early in life, is due in large part to compromised neuropsychological functioning, and is associated with chronic academic or social impairment (or both) across the life span. These conclusions all have profound implications for early identification of and intervention for this disorder in preschool-age children.

## TREATMENT OF ADHD IN EARLY CHILDHOOD

A substantial literature base, including large-scale randomized control trials, has examined interventions for school-age children with ADHD (e.g., MTA Cooperative Group, 1999, 2004). The most common interventions with demonstrated effectiveness are psychotropic medications and behavioral interventions (for a review, see Barkley, 2006). There is little analogous research with preschool-age children. Nonetheless, medication use with young children, particularly methylphenidate hydrochloride (MPH), has increased markedly (e.g., Rappley, 2006). For instance, as noted earlier, data from large and nationally representative groups of children, ages 2 to 4 years, insured by managed care and Medicaid, showed a 1.7- to 3.1-fold increase in MPH use over the previous decade (Zito et al., 2000). A subsequent survey by the Centers for Disease Control and Prevention (2005) indicated that approximately 2.6% of children between 4 and 8 years old are treated with medication for ADHD. The majority of prescriptions written for preschoolers are for stimulants (Zito et al., 2007). Over the 5-year period 2000–2005, younger boys (ages 0–9) showed a 4.0% growth rate in stimulant treatment, a growth rate significantly higher than that for older boys (ages 10–19; 2.3% growth rate; Castle et al., 2007).

Many concerns have emerged regarding the use of psychoactive medications with very young children pertaining to safety and efficacy. Nonetheless, given the exponential increase in medication use with 2- to 4-year-olds, further research was clearly in order. To this end, NIMH funded a large-scale study to evaluate issues of safety and efficacy through controlled research. Specifically, Columbia University and the New York State Psychiatric Institute coordinated a multisite evaluation of MPH in children between 36 and 66 months of age, the Preschool ADHD Treatment Study, or PATS. The results of the PATS indicated that (a) relatively low dosages of MPH led to significant reductions in ADHD symptoms in young children, which were maintained over 10 months for most of the sample (Greenhill et al., 2006; Vitiello et al., 2007); (b) the presence of no or one comorbid disorder (especially ODD) predicted a large treatment response (similar to older children), whereas there was no treatment response for those children with three or more comorbid disorders (Ghuman et al., 2007); (c) a higher percentage of young children relative to elementary school–age children experienced significant adverse events associated with MPH (Wigal et al., 2006); and (d) height and weight growth rates may be reduced for some young children treated with MPH (Swanson et al., 2006).

Given the risk of significant side effects, the use of psychostimulants for treating ADHD in young children must be considered judiciously. Further, there remains broad consensus, echoed by the PATS researchers and consistent with guidelines established by the American Academy of Child and Adolescent Psychiatry and the American Academy of Pediatrics, that behavioral intervention and a structured preschool experience should be the initial course of action before even considering medication use (Gleason et al., 2007; Kollins & Greenhill, 2006; Rappley, 2006). In addition, the long-term advantages of stimulant medication relative to behavioral or psychosocial intervention are unclear (Molina et al., 2009). At this juncture, early implementation of psychosocial intervention appears imperative.

There is considerable empirical support for behavioral parent training and behavioral classroom management as interventions for young children with ADHD (Ghuman, Arnold, & Anthony, 2008; McGoey, Eckert, & DuPaul, 2002; Pelham & Fabiano, 2008). In fact, young children (especially boys) with significant ADHD symptoms may show a greater decrease in externalizing behavior problems as a function of parent training than do young children without ADHD symptoms (Hartman et al., 2003). Sonuga-Barke, Daley, Thompson, Laver-Bradbury, and Weeks (2001) conducted a series of studies that demonstrated the positive impact of parent training on the disruptive and social behavior of young children with ADHD. Similar outcomes have been found in the context of behavioral consultation provided to classroom teachers working with preschoolers with disruptive behaviors, including significant ADHD symptoms (Barkley et al., 2000; Williford & Shelton, 2008). Treatment strategies evaluated in these seminal investigations serve as the critical components of our early intervention program.

# THREE-TIERED INTERVENTION MODEL

Although parent education and other relatively nonintrusive approaches have demonstrated effectiveness, research suggests that there are children who require more intensive interventions because of symptom severity, the presence of significant risk factors, and other variables. In recent years, a tiered model of prevention and intervention has been used successfully as an efficient and effective means of providing the proper type and dosage of treatment (e.g., Chard et al., 2008). Specifically, different dosages or components of intervention are assigned to individuals depending on various factors, including their response to prior interventions (Collins, Murphy, & Bierman, 2004). This model is sometimes referred to as a *stepped-care approach* (e.g., Breslin et al., 1998).

A three-tiered approach to prevention and intervention has its roots in public health. This approach has been used as a classification system for disease prevention for more than 50 years (R. S. Gordon, 1983). In 1952, a working group of the Commission on Chronic Illness proposed a two-tiered approach of primary and secondary prevention, and a third tier (tertiary prevention) was added soon thereafter (Commission on Chronic Illness, 1957). As it has been practiced in the health domain, primary prevention is applied to an entire population before the occurrence of a disease or health problem, with the purpose of reducing or eliminating risk. Examples of primary prevention include immunizations to prevent diseases, fluoride to diminish dental decay, and seat belts to reduce injury during accidents (R. S. Gordon, 1983). Secondary prevention is applied to selected groups when risk factors or disease is recognized but has not yet resulted in a serious affliction. Prevention at the secondary tier includes annual influenza for older individuals, frequent dental visits for those susceptible to dental decay as a result of oral defects, the use of safety goggles for machinists, and airbags in the case of an accident. Tertiary prevention is used for individuals who manifest a disease or have an abnormality that puts them at high risk for disease, with the purpose of preventing further deterioration. Examples include HIV medication to stop viral replication, therapeutic interventions to control hypertension, and root canals to eliminate further tooth infection.

In recent years, the three-tiered model has been applied in education in the areas of behavior and academics. Behavior management historically has been addressed at the classwide and individual levels. In the late 1970s, the importance of prevention at the schoolwide level was recognized, and research studies began to examine the effectiveness of schoolwide interventions for reducing problem behavior (e.g., Mayer & Butterworth, 1979; Sulzer-Azeroff & Mayer, 1986). On the basis of these early efforts, schoolwide positive behavior support (SWPBS), with a three-tiered prevention model, evolved as the leading approach to prevent behavior problems in schools (Sugai & Horner, 2002). This tiered model also has been applied to academics in the form of response to intervention (RtI; Glover & Vaughn, 2010).

Although the SWPBS and RtI models are primarily prevention paradigms, the tiered approach to treatment based on individual response can be applied to early intervention for young children with ADHD. In fact, our early intervention program is a multitiered protocol that individualizes treatment strategies based on individual need and response to prior levels of intervention (for more details, see Chapter 2 of this volume). Because the most intensive treatment resources are provided only to those in need of such services, this model can be time and cost efficient.

## OVERVIEW OF THIS BOOK

The purpose of this book is to provide comprehensive, empirically grounded information on assessment and early intervention for young children with ADHD. Each chapter presents detailed guidelines for assessment and treatment that are data based and practical (i.e., that take into account the inevitable challenges to comprehensive evaluation and treatment in real-world settings). Case illustrations are used throughout to provide examples of early identification and intervention in action.

The organization of this book takes into account several factors. First, we describe the home-based component of early intervention because our experience indicates that most referrals for ADHD will come from primary care physicians and parents, and thus treatment strategies will initially be implemented in the home. Further, some young children do not attend preschool or day care, and intervention would be limited to the home in such cases. Therefore, we present information on home-based intervention before discussing preschool-based strategies. Second, one of the goals of early psychosocial intervention is to delay or avoid pharmacotherapy given the limited data regarding efficacy and safety in early childhood. Thus, medication treatment is not addressed until later in the book. Finally, we present the outcome findings from our early intervention research in the final chapter because we evaluated our program as a comprehensive treatment package (rather than dismantling effects due to each component); this also ensured that the earlier chapters are fully focused on presenting clinically relevant details about intervention.

In Chapter 1, we describe a process for screening and assessing ADHD symptoms in young children with an emphasis on the use of multiple methods (e.g., diagnostic interview, behavior rating scales, direct observations) and multiple respondents (i.e., parent and preschool teacher). The challenges of making an ADHD diagnosis are discussed, along with strategies to best meet those challenges. The emphasis is on using assessment data (e.g., information about behavioral function) to design potentially effective intervention strategies.

Chapter 2 provides an overview of a model for development and implementation of early intervention strategies in home and preschool settings. The key components of the intervention model are detailed briefly, with an emphasis on tiered support as the most cost-efficient strategy. The early intervention model emphasizes addressing all areas in which young children are affected, including problem behavior, preacademic skills, social interactions, and injury prevention. In addition, tips for successful consultation and collaboration are discussed.

The home-based intervention component of the early intervention model is described in Chapter 3. This involves a tiered approach, including (a) group-based parent education, (b) home-based coaching, and (c) assessment-based intervention. Intervention is directed at enhancing behavioral and social functioning. Strategies at each tier are described in detail, along with presentation of data supporting their use.

In Chapter 4, the preschool-based intervention component of the early intervention model is presented. This tiered model includes (a) universal intervention, (b) small-group skills instruction, and (c) assessment-based intervention. This model is directed at enhancing behavioral and social functioning, depending on need. Each intervention tier is described in detail, and data are presented illustrating their use. In addition, broad preschool classroom features (e.g., routines, developmentally appropriate practices) that are essential to the progress of young children with or at risk for ADHD are delineated.

Empirically supported strategies that parents and teachers can use to promote early language, reading, and math skills are described in Chapter 5. Practitioners can teach these strategies in the context of group-based parent education or ongoing consultation by a mental health or special education professional.

In Chapter 6, empirically supported strategies that parents can use to prevent injuries and promote safety in the home setting are described. Details of these strategies are delineated in the context of group-based parent education and ongoing consultation by a mental health or special education professional.

The most common treatment for childhood ADHD is the use of psychostimulant medication (Barkley, 2006). Research studies examining medication in young children with ADHD are described in Chapter 7, including effects on symptomatic behaviors, functional impairment, and possible adverse side effects. Strategies for mental health and special education professionals to help parents and physicians determine whether alternative interventions have been sufficiently implemented and evaluated and then to determine the need for medication and assess both desirable outcomes and side effects are explicated.

Families of children with or at risk for disabilities often experience tremendous stress, which can influence whether and how successful interventions are implemented. In addition, parent–child interactions may be influenced by child behavior. Common family challenges are described in Chapter 8, along with the effects they have on parenting and child outcomes. In addition, current approaches to working with families are discussed. Finally, recommendations are offered to support families and avoid typical problems that arise in relation to having a child with ADHD.

Chapter 9 provides an overview of our early intervention research. In addition, major themes of early intervention are outlined, along with recommendations for future research with this age group. Promising educational and psychological strategies that have been successful for young children with other disorders and that may have application for treatment of young children with ADHD are described.

# 1

# ASSESSMENT AND IDENTIFICATION OF ATTENTION-DEFICIT/ HYPERACTIVITY DISORDER

Given that the behaviors that attention-deficit/hyperactivity disorder (ADHD) comprises (i.e., inattention, impulsivity, high activity) are relatively common among preschool children, comprehensive assessment procedures are needed to make reliable and valid identification decisions. Assessment is important not only in terms of identifying those children requiring services for ADHD but also for making initial and ongoing treatment decisions (Greenhill et al., 2008). Thus, diagnostic measures should focus on relevant symptomatic behaviors and important environmental variables that could account for or maintain those behaviors. Although the diagnostic criteria for ADHD are contextualized within a medical model (i.e., through the *Diagnostic and Statistical Manual of Mental Disorders*, 4th edition, text revision [*DSM–IV–TR*]; American Psychiatric Association, 2000), a comprehensive assessment approach would also provide data regarding environmental factors and possible impairment in academic and social functioning (DuPaul & Stoner, 2003).

To date, most conceptual discussions and empirical studies of ADHD assessment procedures have focused on elementary school–age children (for a review, see Anastopoulos & Shelton, 2001; Pelham, Fabiano, & Massetti,

2005). In recent years, specific measures and strategies have been developed for assessment of emotion and behavior disorders in young children such that diagnosis of ADHD in early childhood has enhanced reliability and validity (Egger, Kondo, & Angold, 2006). Typically, a comprehensive assessment involves diagnostic interviews and behavior rating scales tapping information from parents and teachers. In addition, direct observations of behavior are conducted in the classroom, on the playground, or in analog clinic settings. In most cases, direct tests of attention and impulse control (e.g., Continuous Performance Test) are of limited benefit beyond measures collected in real-world settings. Given the developmental differences between elementary school–age and preschool-age children, as well as the heterogeneity of behavior among young children, it is important to identify reliable and valid assessment methods for this age group that may differ from those used with older children.

The purpose of this chapter is to provide an overview of assessment measures and procedures that can be used to identify and design interventions for young children with ADHD. First, methods to screen for ADHD in young children are described. Screening is critical given that behaviors that may appear to represent ADHD could be symptomatic of another disorder (e.g., autism) or reflect disorganized home or preschool environments. Next, a multi-method assessment approach to identification of ADHD in young children is described. Four core areas of measurement are used: standardized rating scales, structured interviews, direct observations of behavior, and, possibly, direct tests of inattention and impulsivity–hyperactivity (Smith & Corkum, 2007). Key respondents include parents, teachers, and care providers, with an emphasis on assessing both behaviors and environmental variables affecting behavior. Measures to evaluate possible impairments in academic and social functioning are also described. Third, specific challenges to conducting assessments of ADHD in young children are identified, along with strategies to address these challenges. Finally, the use of assessment data (e.g., functional behavioral assessment) to design and evaluate interventions is discussed. Thus, assessment of ADHD does not end with a diagnosis but is used in an ongoing and iterative manner to select and modify intervention strategies.

## SCREENING PROCEDURES

As noted earlier, problems with inattention, impulsive behavior, high activity level, or a combination of these are relatively common among 2- to 5-year-old children, especially in some situations (e.g., unstructured activities in a large group) and at certain times of the day (e.g., end of the day when fatigued). Behaviors that may at first appear to represent ADHD can also be symptomatic of other disorders (e.g., autism, anxiety disorder) or result from exposure to chaotic, disorganized environments (e.g., large preschool classrooms with minimal adult supervision). Thus, when parents, teachers, or care providers indicate that a child exhibits significant problems with attention or impulsivity–hyperactivity, the first step is to collect initial screening data before conducting a more comprehensive behavioral assessment.

The purpose of screening is to identify (a) the need for additional, more costly assessment and (b) whether alternative hypotheses (e.g., other disorders, environmental situation factors) need to be explored before assessing for ADHD. The first step in screening is to ask whoever is reporting the attention and behavior difficulties (e.g., parent, teacher, care provider) to complete a brief questionnaire that requires respondents to report the frequency of ADHD symptomatic behaviors. For example, the Conners Rating Scale (Conners, 2008) contains an ADHD Index that includes the 18 DSM–IV–TR symptoms of ADHD. Normative data for this index are available by age and gender, allowing one to determine the degree to which the frequency of ADHD-related behaviors deviates from other children of the same gender and age. For screening purposes, a relatively liberal threshold (90th percentile) is suggested for determining whether additional assessment of ADHD is warranted. If the ratings for the child's behavior meet or exceed the 90th percentile (i.e., are in the upper 10% of frequency for children's age and gender), then a comprehensive assessment of ADHD (as described later in this chapter) should be conducted. If ratings do not meet this threshold, then a diagnosis of ADHD is unlikely, and the possibility of another disorder or of pursuing environmental modifications (routines, schedules) to reduce behavior and attention problems needs to be considered.

Another screening method would be to ask the person reporting the attention or behavior difficulties to complete ratings of ADHD symptomatic behaviors and determine whether the number of symptoms reported meets DSM–IV–TR criteria. McGoey et al. (2007) adapted the ADHD Rating Scale—IV (DuPaul, Power, Anastopoulos, & Reid, 1998) for the preschool population by modifying items to include examples of behaviors that are more developmentally relevant for this age group. For instance, for the symptom "Does not follow through on instructions and fails to finish tasks," examples are provided such as "Child has difficulty with transitions." Items that are reported to occur "often" or "very often" would count as a symptom being present, whereas those items reported as occurring "not at all" or "sometimes" would represent absent symptoms. The number of endorsed symptoms could be compared with DSM–IV–TR criteria that require six of nine inattention or six of nine hyperactivity–impulsivity symptoms to be present to determine whether additional, more comprehensive assessment is warranted. Of course, one may use a more liberal threshold of four or five symptoms reported as present given that this is a screening stage, and it is sometimes better to allow false positives (i.e., identifying those who will not actually have the disorder after full evaluation) to be assessed further rather than prematurely screening out children who may, in fact, have ADHD.

As noted, problems with inattention, impulse control, and high-frequency physical activity can be manifestations of other developmental or behavioral disorders. When such problems are reported for young children, one hypothesis is that the behaviors could represent a developmental disorder, such as autism. Thus, it is always prudent to simultaneously screen for autism by administering a brief autism questionnaire with parents. In our early intervention research program, we use a two-stage screening process for autism. First, parents are asked questions from the Checklist for Autism in Toddlers (CHAT; Robins, Fein, Barton, & Green, 2001). If the parent answers yes to two or more questions on the CHAT, then the Gilliam Autism Rating Scale (J. E. Gilliam, 1995) is administered. A child receiving an "Autism Quotient" of 121 or higher would require further assessment of autism before any further consideration of possible ADHD. Screening for other possible disorders (i.e., anxiety disorders, depression, oppositional defiant disorder [ODD]) as well as assessment of problematic environmental contexts (e.g., disorganized, poorly controlled preschool classroom) should be part of the comprehensive assessment of ADHD, as described in the next section.

If the screening process indicates that a child may have ADHD in the absence of significant symptoms of autism, then further evaluation is typically warranted. It is important to note that positive screening results do not necessarily mean the child will be diagnosed with ADHD but that there is enough evidence to suggest that further assessment for the disorder is necessary. It is especially important to avoid premature conclusions about the child's diagnostic status on the basis of one or two measures completed by a single respondent. Conclusions based on limited information are not reliable or valid, especially when making a high-stakes decision regarding a child's diagnostic status.

## COMPREHENSIVE ASSESSMENT OF ADHD

A comprehensive assessment of ADHD and related disruptive behavior disorders in young children requires multiple measures obtained across home, preschool, and day care settings using information from multiple respondents. Again, four core methods are used to assess behavior: structured interviews, standardized rating scales, direct observations of behavior, and, possibly, direct tests of attention and hyperactivity–impulsivity (Smith & Corkum, 2007). Assessment data are collected with respect not only to ADHD-related behaviors but also to areas of possible impairment (i.e., academic and social functioning) and environmental factors (e.g., antecedent and consequent events) that could be triggering or maintaining the behaviors of interest. Respondents should include parents, teachers, and care providers (Murray et al., 2007). Finally, a comprehensive assessment should include measures focused on disorders that may be accounting for the apparent ADHD symptoms or may be comorbid with ADHD (e.g., ODD, depression, anxiety disorder).

### Diagnostic Interview With Parent(s)

Parents are key informants in the assessment process because they observe their child's behavior across time and settings and also have direct knowledge of child's medical, family, and treatment histories. Thus, interviewing one or both parents is a critical component of the assessment process. There are three forms of interviews: unstructured, semistructured, and structured. *Unstructured* interviews are essentially open-ended, with the interviewer asking questions in an idiosyncratic order and manner depending on his or her interests and parental responses. Alternatively, *structured* interviews require practitioners to ask questions in a specific manner and sequence following a prescribed format. Often, parents are cued to answer questions in a specific way (e.g., yes or no, choosing from an array of responses on a Likert scale). *Semistructured* interviews typically involve a specific set of questions; however, items may not need to be asked in a set order, or parental responses may be open-ended and not tied to a particular format. Each interview format has relative advantages and disadvantages; however, the use of structured or semistructured interviews is preferred to enhance the reliability and validity of diagnostic decisions (Anastopoulos & Shelton, 2001).

Several structured psychiatric interviews are available (for a detailed discussion of diagnostic interviews, see Barkley, 2006) including the Diagnostic Interview Schedule for Children Version IV (DISC–IV; Shaffer et al., 2000), Diagnostic Interview for Children and Adolescents (Herjanic & Reich, 1982), and Schedule for Affective Disorders and Schizophrenia for School-Age Children (Orvaschel & Puig-Antich, 1994). We have used the DISC–IV in our early intervention studies because interview items are tied directly to the *DSM–IV–TR* criteria. The interview can be administered and scored via computer, and an early childhood version is available. The interview involves asking parents to report the presence or absence of each ADHD symptomatic behavior, the degree to which these symptoms impair child functioning in academic skills or social performance, whether the symptoms are present across more than one setting, and whether symptomatic behaviors have occurred at a high frequency over at least a 6-month period. In addition, parents are asked about behaviors that are symptomatic of other disruptive behavior (i.e., ODD and conduct disorder [CD]) and internalizing (e.g., separation anxiety disorder, depression) disorders. The primary advantage of this structured interview format is that responses are scored to indicate whether diagnostic criteria for ADHD or other disorders are met. Further, questions are asked in a standardized fashion that can minimize potential bias and variability in information obtained across parents (i.e., increases reliability of diagnostic decisions). As such, a structured interview such as the DISC–IV is useful for research purposes in which it is critical to follow standardized procedures across participants. The primary disadvantages are that the interview takes at least 60 minutes to complete, and there is limited flexibility for interviewers to improvise questions or probe parent responses.

Semistructured interviews may be the best option for clinical purposes because they prompt parents to provide information about *DSM–IV–TR* symptoms while allowing interviewers some flexibility to ask open-ended questions and follow up on parental responses as necessary. Barkley and Murphy (2006) provided a semistructured diagnostic interview that can be administered with parents that covers all of the relevant *DSM–IV–TR* diagnostic categories and also asks about the child's medical, treatment, and family histories. In fact, the questions about history from this interview can be used to supplement a structured diagnostic interview when the latter is used (note that most structured diagnostic interviews do not cover medical, treatment, or family histories). This semistructured interview may take less time to complete because the interviewer has the option to skip sections or specific questions if they are not relevant. Unfortunately, this semistructured interview is not available for computer administration and must be completed by hand.

Assessment of older children with ADHD typically includes a teacher interview focused on symptomatic behaviors, classroom functioning, and prior or current intervention strategies (DuPaul & Stoner, 2003). If a young child is in a preschool or day care setting, then the preschool teacher or care provider can also be interviewed regarding the presence or absence of ADHD symptoms as well as behaviors related to other disorders (e.g., autism, depression, ODD). Of even greater importance, teachers or care providers can report on antecedent and consequent events that trigger or reinforce the target behaviors, respectively. Interviewing teachers and parents about behavioral function and environmental events is discussed further in the section Going Beyond Diagnosis: Linking Assessment to Intervention.

### Behavior Rating Scales

Standardized behavior rating scales provide important information about the degree to which children's symptomatic behaviors deviate from behaviors of peers of the same age and gender, at least from the point of view of parents and teachers. It is important to obtain ratings on at least one broadband rating scale and one narrowband rating scale. Broadband questionnaires include items related to a variety of externalizing and internalizing disorders. These measures provide critical data that can help to determine whether behaviors originally thought to represent ADHD might alternatively be manifestations of another disorder or could indicate that behaviors symptomatic of other disorders are occurring along with ADHD. Commonly used broadband questionnaires for the early childhood population include the Child Behavior Checklist (Achenbach & Rescorla, 2000) and corollary Teacher Report Form (Achenbach & Rescorla, 2000), as well as parent and teacher versions of the Behavior Assessment System for Children—2 (BASC–2; Reynolds & Kamphaus, 2002). A broadband measure that includes items directly tied to *DSM–IV–TR* criteria for a variety of disorders is the Early Childhood Inventory—4 (Gadow & Sprafkin, 1997). The popular Conners Rating Scales (Conners, 2008) provides good coverage of externalizing disorder symptoms (including ADHD); however, it includes limited internalizing disorder items. All of these questionnaires have impeccable psychometric properties and are good choices for inclusion in an assessment protocol (for a review, see Pelham, Fabiano, & Massetti, 2005). Thus, the selection of one of these instruments is based primarily on practitioner preference.

Narrowband rating scales are brief measures that tap parent and teacher perceptions of ADHD-related behaviors. Typically, these questionnaires include items that are directly tied to the ADHD symptoms as described in *DSM–IV–TR*. Examples include the ADHD Rating Scale—IV—Preschool Version (McGoey et al., 2007), ADHD Symptoms Rating Scale (ADHD–SRS; Phillips, Greenson, Collett, & Gimpel, 2002), and the Conners Teacher Rating Scale—Revised for Preschoolers (Purpura & Lonigan, 2009). As is the case for broadband measures, all of these ADHD-specific scales have adequate psychometric properties and relatively current normative data. Thus, practitioner preference is the basis for selecting one from among the available questionnaires.

## Direct Observations of Behavior

Although diagnostic interviews and behavior rating scales are important components of a comprehensive ADHD evaluation protocol, data obtained from these measures are inherently biased by the perceptions of parents and teachers. Thus, additional, more objective indices are useful. Practitioners, trained paraprofessionals, or students can conduct direct observations of children's behavior in home, preschool, or analog clinic settings (DeWolfe, Byrne, & Bawden, 2000). Presumably, the perceptions of external observers are less subject to biases than those of parents and teachers, especially when structured coding systems are used. Structured coding systems provide operational definitions of key behaviors as well as standardized time periods or intervals in which behavior is observed. Given that the symptomatic behaviors of ADHD occur in a variety of settings and may manifest differently across environments, ideally, observations would be conducted in several venues, including structured and unstructured situations.

Behavior observation systems that have been used successfully in assessing young children with ADHD and related disorders include the classroom observation code (Abikoff, Gittelman-Klein, & Klein, 1977), Early Screening Project (ESP) coding system (Feil, Walker, & Severson, 1995), and the parent–child interaction observation code (Strain, Steele, Ellis, & Timm, 1982). In addition, DeWolfe and colleagues (2000) developed a clinic-based observation code focused on task engagement, play duration, and activity shifts that discriminates well between preschoolers with and without ADHD. The classroom observation code has been used widely in ADHD research studies including investigations with young children. The behaviors coded in this system (see Table 1.1) are particularly relevant for structured preschool classroom situations, such as circle time or other activities that require children to sit still, pay attention, and wait their turn. Observations are conducted for 15 to 30 minutes, with each minute divided into three 15-second observe, 5-second record intervals. Following the completion of the observation session, the percentage of intervals in which each behavior occurred can be calculated.

The ESP coding system can be used for observations of behavior in unstructured preschool settings (e.g., free play), as specific categories of play and social behavior are included (see Table 1.1). As with the classroom observation code, sessions last between 15 and 30 minutes with three 15-second observa-

TABLE 1.1
Direct Observation Systems and Coding Categories

| Observation system | Coding categories |
| --- | --- |
| Classroom observation code (Abikoff et al., 1977) | Interference, solicitation, off-task, minor motor movements, gross motor movements |
| Early Screening Project coding system (Walker et al., 1995) | Negative verbal, negative physical, disruptive behavior, off-task, activity change, type of play (solitary, parallel), positive social |
| Parent–child interaction observation (Strain et al., 1982) | *Parent behaviors:* Type of command (alpha, beta), positive response, negative response<br>*Child behaviors:* noncompliance, positive social, negative social, appropriate nonsocial, inappropriate nonsocial |

tion intervals per minute. Data are collected for both the target student and randomly selected peers of the same gender to provide a local normative comparison. This comparison of target student and peer observation data is helpful in determining the degree to which the target child's behavior deviates from classmates as well as providing a gauge of the overall teacher management of the setting. In fact, it is a good idea to include peer data for structured classroom observations as well because this information may be helpful in determining whether a child's ADHD behaviors stand out from the classroom norm or represent a broader, classwide behavior management problem.

It is not always possible to observe children's behavior in their homes, but data regarding parent–child interactions are helpful for both diagnostic and treatment planning purposes. Negative interactions between parents and children characterize not only the family situations of young children with ADHD but also coercive interchanges that may promote the development of child antisocial behavior (Patterson, Reid, & Dishion, 1992). In our early intervention work, we conducted observations of parent and child behavior during dinnertime, a situation that occurs in most homes and that may be a time when problematic interactions occur. The parent–child observation code includes several categories of parent and child behavior (see Table 1.1) observed across a 20- to 30-minute session. Each minute is divided into three 15-second observations, 5-second record intervals, allowing for calculation of the percentage of intervals in which each behavior occurs. Practitioners could also use this system to examine microexchanges between parents and children wherein the probability of specific child or parent behaviors in any interval can be determined on the basis of behavior that occurred in preceding or subsequent intervals. Stated differently, one could examine the chain of parent–child behavior interchanges across intervals. These data could be helpful in developing hypotheses about the function of child behavior and ultimately aid in selecting possible intervention strategies (see Chapter 3, this volume).

### Clinic-Based Tests of Attention and Hyperactivity–Impulsivity

There is some controversy in the ADHD field as to whether clinic-based tests of attention and hyperactivity–impulsivity provide useful diagnostic and intervention planning data. Some researchers (Barkley, 2006; DuPaul & Stoner, 2003) have asserted that clinic-based tests are of limited value given that performance is assessed on contrived tasks in settings that do not resemble the "real world" of homes and classrooms. These tests are viewed to have limited external validity, and practitioners are advised that it is better to use time and resources to gather data about children's behavior in natural settings. Alternatively, others (DeWolfe, Byrne, & Bawden, 1999; Mahone, Pillion, & Hiemenz, 2001; Mahone, Pillion, Hoffman, Hernandez, & Denckla, 2005;

Tandon, Si, Beiden, & Luby, 2009) have argued that newly developed measures can provide data about attention and impulsivity that are helpful supplements to information gathered through interviews and rating scales.

Clinic-based tests of attention and/or hyperactivity–impulsivity include the Auditory Continuous Performance Test for Preschoolers (Mahone, Pillion, & Hiemenz, 2001), Conners Continuous Performance Test—Kiddie Version (Conners, 2001), and the Gordon Diagnostic System (M. Gordon, 1996). Although the developers of these measures provide empirical support for the reliability and validity of test data, the question remains whether the information derived is worth the time, effort, and resources compared with what can be obtained from interviews, rating scales, and direct observations. From our perspective, children and families are better served if practitioners use the time they would have devoted to such testing to conduct observations of children's behaviors as well as environmental antecedent and consequent events in home and preschool settings. These data will not only be helpful in the context of diagnosis and assessment but will also provide critical information that can be used for intervention planning purposes (see "Going Beyond Diagnosis: Link Assessment to Intervention"). There is no evidence that clinic-based tests of attention and hyperactivity–impulsivity are useful for treatment planning efforts.

### Screening for Alternative or Comorbid Disorders

An important step in the comprehensive assessment of ADHD is to collect data that shed light on alternative hypotheses for behaviors that appear symptomatic of this disorder. For example, young children with autism may display problems attending to activities, may respond impulsively, or may engage in high rates of motor activity (American Psychiatric Association, 2000). Although these behaviors may first appear to be symptomatic of ADHD, they could be manifestations of a pervasive developmental disorder. Thus, measures should be included to screen for and rule out other disorders that may be mistakenly labeled ADHD (see Table 1.2). Symptomatic behaviors of other

TABLE 1.2
Possible Alternative and Comorbid Disorders

| Disorders with symptom overlap with ADHD | Possible comorbid disorders |
|---|---|
| Autism, Asperger's disorder, conduct disorder, cyclothymia, dysthymia, generalized anxiety disorder, major depression, oppositional defiant disorder, pediatric-onset bipolar disorder | Conduct disorder, generalized anxiety disorder, learning disabilities, major depression, oppositional defiant disorder, separation anxiety disorder, tic disorders |

disorders can be reviewed as part of the diagnostic interview with parents and also assessed with broadband behavior ratings. To the extent that interview responses and/or questionnaire subscale data indicate elevated symptoms of other disorders, further evaluation is warranted before reaching any diagnostic conclusions.

ADHD is a disorder that rarely occurs in isolation, at least in most clinic-based studies (Barkley, 2006). In fact, several externalizing and internalizing disorders can be comorbid with ADHD (see Table 1.2). Once again, diagnostic interview and broadband rating scale data are helpful in identifying possible co-occurring or comorbid conditions that may require additional assessment. Of course, the presence of co-occurring disorders not only complicates the diagnostic decision-making process but also introduces complexity into intervention planning. Specifically, practitioners must help families and teachers to prioritize target behaviors for intervention among the symptoms of two or more disorders.

### Assessment of Academic and Social Functioning

By definition, a diagnosis of ADHD requires children to show either academic or social impairment as a function of their symptomatic behaviors (American Psychiatric Association, 2000). Stated differently, it is not sufficient to demonstrate that a child exhibits the requisite number of inattentive or hyperactive–impulsive symptoms; the child must also show some functional deficits in relation to these symptoms. Impairment in functioning can be assessed in at least three ways (Healey, Miller, Castelli, Marks, & Halperin, 2008). First, parents and teachers can be asked about possible impairment as part of the diagnostic interview. For example, many structured interviews include an item asking parents whether the symptoms they have observed have caused problems with academic or social functioning. Of course, this is a very general indicator of functional impairment that does not provide precise data and may have rather limited reliability and validity.

A second and more precise method of documenting functional impairment is through parent and teacher ratings. Practitioners can ask respondents to complete a broad-based impairment rating, such as the Impairment Rating Scale (Fabiano et al., 2006) or the Children's Problem Checklist (Healey et al., 2008), or more specific ratings of key areas, such as the Social Skills Improvement Systems Rating Scales (Gresham & Elliott, 2008) and the Academic Competence Evaluation Scale (DiPerna & Elliott, 2000). Information from these scales can delineate the degree to which children show impairment in these areas relative to a normative population.

The final and most precise method for assessing academic and social functioning is to use direct measures in each area. Norm-referenced tests of early language, math, and reading abilities, such as the Bracken Basic Concept Scale—Revised (Bracken, 1998), provide age-appropriate information about early academic skills. Criterion-referenced tests specific to early academic skills may be of even greater value given that the data obtained may translate more directly to instructional strategies. For reading and language, Phonological Awareness Literacy Screening (Invernizzi, Sullivan, Meier, & Swank, 2004) and Dynamic Indicators of Basic Early Literacy Skills (Kaminski & Good, 1996) have good psychometric properties with the early childhood population. Fewer measures are available for early math skills, but some recently devised instruments include the Early Numeracy Skills Assessment (Sokol, 2002) and the Preschool Numeracy Indicators (Floyd, Hojnoski, & Key, 2006; Hojnoski, Silberglitt, & Floyd, 2009).

Direct assessment of social skills and peer status is less straightforward. Behavioral observations of children's behavior in unstructured or playground settings can be conducted to document the frequency of positive and negative social behaviors relative to peers (see the prior discussion of direct observations of behavior). Although seemingly objective, observations of social behavior are limited because data are available only for a small cross-section of time. This is especially problematic for assessment of infrequent behaviors, such as physical aggression. Assessment of peer social status typically involves collection of sociometric measures in which children report on who they like and dislike. Such information may be helpful in documenting children's acceptance or rejection by peers; however, these are sensitive data to obtain because educators and parents may consider it inappropriate to ask children to judge their relationship with others (particularly to identify peers they do not prefer) and thus are rarely used outside of research investigations.

## INTERPRETATION OF ASSESSMENT DATA

After comprehensive assessment data are collected, practitioners must then interpret the data to render a diagnostic decision and develop an intervention plan. With respect to the diagnosis of ADHD, the primary approach is to follow *DSM–IV–TR* criteria as closely as possible (see Exhibit 1.1). The first step is to determine how many of the behavioral symptoms of ADHD are reported to occur within both symptom categories (i.e., inattention and hyperactivity–impulsivity). There are two ways to conduct symptom counts. One is to tally the number of symptomatic behaviors reported to occur on a frequent basis by parents on the diagnostic interview. A second way is to tally the number of symptomatic behaviors reported to occur often or very often on a narrowband parent or teacher rating of ADHD symptoms. Then symptom counts can be compared with *DSM* criteria stipulating a minimum of six

## EXHIBIT 1.1

Steps to Diagnostic Decision Making

1. Determine the number of behavioral symptoms of inattention and hyperactivity–impulsivity on the basis of parent diagnostic interview and/or symptom counts from parent and teacher behavior ratings.
2. Determine whether inattentive or hyperactive–impulsive behaviors deviate significantly from age and gender norms using parent and teacher behavior rating scales.
3. Determine whether there is clinically significant impairment in academic or social functioning based on parent–teacher rating scales, and/or direct measures of functioning.
4. Establish whether ADHD symptoms and associated impairment is displayed in two or more settings on the basis of direct observations, parent–teacher ratings, and direct measures of functioning.
5. Identify whether purported ADHD symptoms are better accounted for by another disorder (e.g., autism) on the basis of diagnostic interview and parent–teacher behavior ratings.
6. Evaluate whether environmental events and contextual factors (e.g., lack of structure and clear, consistent management in a preschool classroom) can better account for what appear to be behaviors symptomatic of ADHD.

*Note.* ADHD = attention-deficit/hyperactivity disorder.

of nine inattention or six of nine hyperactivity–impulsivity symptoms (or both). Of course, given that many young children will exhibit inattentive or hyperactive–impulsive behaviors on occasion, it is also important to determine whether the frequency and severity of these behaviors actually deviates from expected developmental levels. Currently, the best way to determine this is by comparing children's scores on parent and teacher behavior rating scales with population-based norms for age and gender. If scores are in the 93rd percentile or higher for age and gender, then symptoms are considered clinically significant (Anastopoulos & Shelton, 2001; Barkley, 2006).

The second *DSM–IV–TR* criterion to consider is whether there is clear evidence of clinically significant impairment in social or academic functioning associated with the ADHD-related behaviors. For the social domain, practitioners should examine scores on a parent-completed social skills rating scale (e.g., Social Skills Improvement System Rating Scales; Gresham & Elliott, 2008) to see whether interpersonal difficulties exceed levels expected for a child's age and gender. For this purpose, we recommend a slightly more liberal cutpoint of scores at or above the 90th percentile, meaning that social difficulties are in the upper 10% for a child's age and gender. If the child is in a preschool or day care setting, then social skills ratings should also be obtained from teachers or day care providers. In fact, teacher ratings of social skills should take precedence over parent ratings given that teachers have a greater opportunity to observe children interacting with peers.

Assessing possible impairment in the academic domain among preschoolers is challenging because many children at that age are not exposed to academic instruction, and floor effects are expected on standardized achievement tests. *Floor effects* refer to situations in which children's scores gather at the bottom of a distribution of scores because the test is too difficult for that group of children. Most norm-referenced, standardized achievement tests are designed to test academic skills of children in grades K through 12. As a result, many preschoolers may not be able to answer more than a few questions on each subtest. Thus, standardized achievement tests, at least those typically used for evaluating elementary and secondary school students, have limited value for assessment of young children. Alternatively, standardized measures of preacademic skills (e.g., Bracken Basic Concept Scale—Revised) have been developed for use with young children. Scores that are more than 1 standard deviation below age norms can indicate significant impairment in the development of prereading, premath, and other school readiness skills—that is, the child's performance on early academic skills falls in approximately the lowest 16% compared with his or her peers.

A third *DSM–IV–TR* criterion to consider is the requirement that impairment due to ADHD-related behaviors is reported in two or more settings. Stated differently, assessment data should demonstrate that ADHD symptomatic behaviors and associated impairment are cross-situational. Thus, practitioners can look at narrowband symptom and social skills ratings across home, preschool, and day care settings. To the degree that parents and teachers are consistent in reporting significant levels of symptoms and impairment, this criterion will be met. If such ratings are discrepant across settings, then this criterion is not met, and the diagnosis of ADHD becomes questionable. The presence of symptoms across settings is important because it supports the diagnosis of ADHD, rather than simply the presence of problem behavior resulting from environmental variables (e.g., lack of structure) that exist in a single setting. Divergence in rater scores also can reflect different tolerance levels for problem behavior; hence, a diagnosis of ADHD should be carefully considered. Direct observations of behavior in home and preschool settings can help in the case of discrepant ratings by showing whether ADHD-related behaviors and associated impairments are present or absent in a given environment. In general, parent interview and ratings of ADHD symptoms should be weighed more heavily because of their presumed greater familiarity with their children's behaviors. Alternatively, teacher ratings of social and academic impairment should be considered foremost given teachers' greater opportunity to observe interpersonal interactions and the development of preacademic skills.

The next *DSM–IV–TR* criterion to consider is whether the putative ADHD symptoms are not better accounted for by other disorders (e.g., autism, ODD, and separation anxiety disorder). Three components of the comprehensive assessment can be used in considering this criterion. Parent responses to diagnostic interview items surveying symptoms of various disorders other than ADHD can be tallied to see whether criteria are met for these disorders. This is particularly critical with respect to autism symptoms that may better account for children's attention and behavior difficulties. Of course, the fact that diagnostic criteria are met for another disorder (other than autism or schizophrenia) does not necessarily mean that a child does not also have ADHD given the relatively high rate of comorbidity in this population.

A second component of the assessment to consider in relation to whether other disorders may better account for the apparent ADHD symptoms is a broadband behavior rating scale (e.g., Child Behavior Checklist) completed by parents and teachers. Typically, broadband ratings include separate subscales that correspond with various disorders. For example, the BASC–2 includes subscales that tap behavioral symptoms of several disorders, including ODD and CD. Thus, practitioners can compare children's subscale scores to age and gender norms using a 93rd percentile cutoff for clinical significance. Those subscales that meet or exceed the 93rd percentile may indicate the presence of that particular disorder, especially when (a) diagnostic interview responses are positive for that disorder and (b) parent and teacher ratings are in agreement (i.e., indicating cross-situational consistency).

Given the particular interest in ruling out autism in the preschool age group, a third component to consider is parent ratings on an autism questionnaire. If these ratings meet established cut points for the presence of autism, then further assessment of this disorder is warranted before making any decisions about an ADHD diagnosis. The fact that ratings meet screening criteria for autism does not necessarily mean that the child has autism and does not have ADHD but that further evaluation is warranted. If after further evaluation a diagnosis of autism is appropriate, then intervention for behaviors associated with this disorder (e.g., language deficits, problems with joint attention, social withdrawal) takes top priority, and the presence or absence of ADHD is a secondary concern. Alternatively, if autism is ruled out with further assessment, then ADHD can be reconsidered.

In addition to considering *DSM* criteria for ADHD, it is important to evaluate alternative hypotheses for what appear to be symptomatic behaviors. In particular, environmental events and contextual factors may elicit inattentive, impulsive, and/or highly active behaviors in young children in the absence of ADHD. For example, children in poorly managed or chaotic classroom or home environments may appear distractible, disruptive, and physically active because of the lack of structure and clear behavioral expectations in that setting. From a behavioral perspective, antecedent events (e.g., unclear task demands) may set the occasion for inattentive, disruptive behavior, and consequent events (e.g., teacher attention to inappropriate actions) may maintain these behaviors over time. Direct observations, especially in the context of a functional behavioral assessment, can provide data that are helpful in examining whether environmental events may be contributing to challenging behavior on a classwide basis or in the home. In a poorly managed, disorganized environment, it is difficult to ascertain whether children's behaviors represent a disruptive behavior disorder such as ADHD or whether these behaviors are simply a manifestation of that environment. The most prudent course of action, then, is to work with teachers or parents to change the structure and management of the environment to see whether individual children continue to exhibit challenging behaviors after changes are made.

Another possible environmental precursor to inattentive and hyperactive–impulsive behavior in young children is the experience of a significant change, usually negative, in their lives. Sometimes when children experience a traumatic event (e.g., death of a parent, sibling, or family pet), they may temporarily exhibit problems with concentration, behavior control, or both. More likely, they may show signs of stress that can include anxiety-induced distractibility, fidgetiness, and diminished task productivity. These reactions may be temporary or may be associated with more chronic difficulties, such as posttraumatic stress disorder. In any case, traumatic events or significant life events may be associated with some behaviors that mimic ADHD, but such events do not lead to a "true" manifestation of this disorder (Barkley, 2006).

## CHALLENGES TO ASSESSMENT OF ADHD IN YOUNG CHILDREN

In the absence of a single, objective "test" for ADHD, making conclusions about this diagnosis can be challenging under the best of circumstances but is even more challenging when assessing young children for several reasons. First, children in the preschool years exhibit a wide range of behaviors depending on who they are with and the variables (e.g., activities, structure) within the setting. This inherent heterogeneity of behavior makes it difficult to discern whether apparent problems with attention or hyperactivity–impulsivity represent a disorder (i.e., behavior that is substantially deviant from norms for children's age and gender) or if these are simply behaviors that lie at the extreme end of the range of typical behavior (i.e., represent the tail end of the natural distribution of these behaviors in the population). Campbell (2002) offered guidelines for making this diagnostic discrimination. Specifically, practitioners must identify a combination of problem behaviors that occur together at a significantly higher frequency and severity compared with similar-age children, and these problems must occur for a sufficiently long duration to make them distinct from an adjustment to a life event (e.g., birth of sibling) or a developmental transition (e.g., entry into preschool). Further, problem behaviors should be present across settings and adult relationships and must impair the development of typical skills and abilities.

A second, related challenge to diagnostic assessment of ADHD in young children is the possible attenuation of behavior difficulties with development (Loughran, 2003). A series of studies conducted by Campbell and colleagues (e.g., Campbell & Ewing, 1990; Campbell, Ewing, Breaux, & Szumowski, 1986) in the 1980s and 1990s appeared to indicate that approximately 50% of preschoolers with apparent ADHD "outgrew" their disorder when assessed later in elementary school. Stated differently, these children did not truly have ADHD, particularly given that it is almost always a chronic condition that persists across development (see Barkley, Murphy, & Fischer, 2008). Rather, some young children may exhibit inattention and/or hyperactivity–impulsivity for a year or two during early childhood, perhaps as a manifestation of developmental differences or delays. Thus, it is always important to use caution in applying the diagnosis of ADHD with young children because a substantial proportion of them will not continue to exhibit this disorder into elementary school. It may be helpful to refer to such children as being *at risk for ADHD* rather than applying the diagnostic label without qualifiers. It is important to note that more recent longitudinal studies using current diagnostic criteria and assessment measures indicate that most young children meeting diagnostic criteria for ADHD will persist with significant symptoms through childhood and adolescence (e.g., Lahey et al., 2004). Nevertheless, in many cases, cautionary labels, such as *at risk for ADHD*, should be considered when working with young children whose difficulties may be relatively ephemeral.

A final challenge to assessment of ADHD in young children is that for most children, only limited information is available regarding behavior outside of the home setting. Some children do not attend preschool or child care programs. Even children who attend preschool may only do so a few days per week and for limited amounts of time. Preschool teachers and day care providers can contribute information as part of the assessment, but they may have limited opportunities to observe child behavior across a variety of contexts and for a sufficient period of time. Thus, parents will be the primary, and in some cases sole, informants regarding ADHD symptoms. Unfortunately, this reliance on parental report may lead to unreliable or invalid diagnostic decisions; studies have shown that sole use of maternal report may lead to overidentification (Gimpel & Kuhn, 2000) or underidentification (Maniadaki, Sonuga-Barke, Kakouros, & Karaba, 2007) of ADHD. Even when teacher ratings are available, correlations between parent and teacher ratings of ADHD symptoms are relatively low (i.e., $r < .30$), indicating that child behavior varies considerably across settings (Murray et al., 2007).

Although diagnostic and assessment decisions related to ADHD in young children can be challenging, several strategies can help practitioners meet these challenges in an effective fashion. First, psychometrically sound assessment measures that include normative data for young children should be used. Since the late 1990s, many teacher and parent behavior rating scales have been developed to assess ADHD symptoms in young children (see "Comprehensive Assessment of ADHD" earlier in the chapter). Care should be taken to choose the measures that best represent the population from which target children are drawn. For example, a rating scale that includes normative data from an ethnically diverse population should be used when assessing children from non-White backgrounds.

A second strategy to enhance the assessment process is to use multiple measures rather than relying on a single index to make diagnostic decisions. As discussed previously, there is no single evaluation method to identify children with ADHD, especially when children are in a developmental phase that involves rapid changes in functioning that vary considerably across children. Reliable and valid diagnostic and treatment decisions are more likely to occur when multiple respondents (i.e., parents and teachers) and multiple methods (i.e., parent interview; behavior rating scales completed by parents and teachers; direct observations; possibly, clinic-based tests) are used to gauge behavior across settings. The latter may be particularly helpful in situations in which teacher ratings are not available.

Third, it is critical that an evaluation of ADHD focus on functional impairments that might be associated with symptomatic behaviors. As we have noted, given that many young children may exhibit high activity, short attention span, and/or impulsive behavior, the degree to which these behaviors lead to impairment is what differentiates children with ADHD from their typically developing peers. Further, including an objective measure of impairment can reduce diagnosis of ADHD in preschoolers by 46% to 77% over assessments that simply consider the presence or absence of symptoms (Healey et al., 2008). A comprehensive evaluation includes assessment of social, preacademic, and family functioning. If significant impairments are identified and these deficits appear linked to ADHD-related behaviors, then practitioners are on firmer ground when rendering a diagnosis. To the extent that functioning is not impaired, a diagnosis of ADHD is not warranted (American Psychiatric Association, 2000).

Cross-sectional (e.g., DuPaul et al., 2001) and longitudinal (e.g., Lahey et al., 2004) investigations have documented acute and chronic difficulties experienced by young children with ADHD. Thus, it is clear that inclusion criteria used in these studies identify a group of children who are at immediate and long-term risk for behavioral and academic difficulties. These investigations employed a multiple-method, multiple-respondent approach to identifying participants, which included diagnostic interviews with parents, behavior ratings by parents and teachers, and an effort to exclude competing hypotheses (e.g., autism) for apparent ADHD symptoms. These data provide empirical support for using the assessment methods described in this chapter.

Despite the use of these assessment strategies, diagnostic decisions about ADHD in young children should be made with appropriate caution. In fact, one option is to use the phrase *at risk for ADHD* when describing young children who meet diagnostic criteria but for whom assessment data may be incomplete (e.g., no teacher ratings are available) or marginally significant (e.g., child's symptoms are in the mild range in terms of severity and impairment). This phrase communicates that a child's behavior deviates sufficiently from that of his or her same-age peers to place that child at risk for a variety of difficulties, but it also indicates that a firm conclusion about diagnostic status awaits further child development (e.g., after the child enters elementary school).

## ASSESSMENT CASE EXAMPLE

Jason D., a 3-year-old, White, non-Hispanic boy, was referred to our early intervention program by his preschool center director because of concerns about his very high activity level, problems attending to preschool rules and activities, and difficulties getting along with peers and teachers. Jason was in a full-year preschool program and attended the center 4 days per week. Ms. D., his 22-year-old mother, reported similar challenging behaviors for Jason in the home setting. At the time of the referral, Jason's parents were separated, and he was living with his mother and older brother. Both Ms. D. and Jason's father were high school graduates and employed.

Ms. D. and Jason's primary preschool teacher completed the Conners Rating Scales. Both parent and teacher ratings placed Jason's ADHD- and ODD-related behaviors beyond the 98th percentile for his gender and age. Specifically, he obtained standard scores of 90 (both parent and teacher) on the Oppositional subscale and standard scores of 88 (parent) and 81 (teacher) on the ADHD Index. A clinical interview with Ms. D. using the DISC-IV indicated that Jason displayed all nine inattentive and all nine hyperactive–impulsive symptoms from the *DSM-IV* ADHD criteria. These behaviors were reported to occur at a high frequency, to be chronic (i.e., duration of at least 1 year), and to cause impairment across home and preschool settings. In addition, Ms. D. reported that Jason displayed all eight behavioral symptoms of ODD on a frequent basis. Thus, clinical interview data were consistent with diagnoses of ADHD—combined type and ODD.

Jason was reported to exhibit one symptom of CD (i.e., physically cruel to people) but did not meet the full criteria for this disorder. Ms. D.'s responses to the Checklist for Autism in Toddlers ruled out autism symptoms and indicated that no further assessment of developmental disability was warranted. Further, Jason obtained low-average-range standard scores (low 90s) on the verbal and nonverbal clusters of the Differential Ability Scales. Thus, his challenging behaviors did not appear to be related to cognitive deficits. A brief (20-minute) observation of Jason's behavior in his preschool classroom was conducted using the classroom observation code (Abikoff et al., 1977). These data were collected to ascertain Jason's behavior in a structured situation (e.g., group circle time). Data were also gathered for a randomly selected comparison peer of the same gender. During this observation, Jason displayed relatively high rates of off-task behavior and noncompliance. Specifically, he was off-task during 18% of the intervals relative to only 8% of intervals for the comparison peer. In similar fashion, he displayed noncompliant behavior during 5% of the intervals, whereas the comparison peer did not display any noncompliant behavior. Jason was not observed to be physically aggressive during the structured setting. An additional 15-minute observation using the ESP coding system (Feil et al., 1995) was conducted during free play on a playground just outside of the classroom. Jason showed lower levels of positive social engagement (15% of intervals) compared with a randomly selected peer (45% of intervals) and exhibited more negative verbal (13% vs. 1% for peer) and physical (5% vs. 0% for peer) behavior toward classmates.

Assessment data were consistent in identifying chronic, cross-situational, and impairing behavioral symptoms of ADHD for Jason. Competing hypotheses (e.g., CD, autism, cognitive deficits) for these behaviors were also ruled out. Further, both parent and teacher reports indicate behaviors consistent with ODD. Thus, Jason appears to meet diagnostic criteria for ADHD—combined type and ODD. As a result, his mother and teacher agreed to participate in our early intervention program in an effort to reduce his challenging behaviors and enhance his behavioral and social functioning. Additional assessment data were collected to aid in intervention design, as described in the next section.

## GOING BEYOND DIAGNOSIS: LINKING ASSESSMENT TO INTERVENTION

The assessment process for children suspected of having ADHD does not end with a diagnostic decision but continues as intervention strategies are selected and implemented. In fact, in many ways, intervention selection and evaluation are the most important aspects of the assessment process, perhaps more critical from a clinical perspective than arriving at a diagnosis (DuPaul & Stoner, 2003). Assessment data help with treatment selection in several ways. First, data directly related to intervention design should be collected contemporaneously with data gathered for diagnostic purposes. For example, during direct observations of behavior, rather than simply taking frequency counts of ADHD-related behaviors (e.g., off task), practitioners can note environmental events that precede or trigger behaviors, as well as those events that follow and may serve as consequences to specific behaviors. In such fashion, information helpful for both diagnosis and intervention design can be obtained simultaneously.

A major decision, particularly with respect to treatment of ADHD, is whether psychotropic medication (see Chapter 7) should be prescribed. Although stimulant medications (e.g., methylphenidate) lead to significant reductions in ADHD symptoms for many children, findings suggest that preschoolers may be more prone to adverse side effects than older children and that parents of young children find pharmacotherapy less acceptable than do parents of older children and adolescents with ADHD (Greenhill et al., 2006; Swanson et al., 2006). Thus, the general preference is to avoid or delay the use of medication, particularly for the preschool age group (see Chapter 7). Data regarding the severity of ADHD symptoms and associated impairment as well as response to prior intervention can be used as a guide for medication decisions. Specifically, medication would be considered as a first-line treatment only for those young children who display highly frequent and severe symptoms of the disorder (i.e., at least 2 standard deviations above the mean for age and gender) along with severe deficits in academic or social skills (i.e., at least 2 standard deviations below the mean for the child's age). Psychosocial, educational, and home safety interventions (as described in subsequent chapters) would be preferred first-line treatments in all but the most severe cases.

Beyond the general decision as to whether medication is included, assessment data can guide more specific intervention decisions. The most prominent example of assessment-based intervention is the design of intervention strategies based on functional assessment (T. S. Watson & Steege, 2003). A functional assessment is designed to identify those environmental events that precede or follow a behavior that appear to be functionally related to the display of that behavior. In subsequent chapters, the specific steps involved in functional assessment are described in greater detail for both home (see Chapter 3) and preschool (see Chapter 4) settings. In general, a functional assessment involves gathering descriptive information from parents or teachers regarding possible antecedent and consequent events that may be eliciting and maintaining specific target behaviors, respectively. In some cases, experimental analyses may be conducted to manipulate consequences directly to determine behavioral function. The final stage of a functional assessment involves testing an intervention that elicits or reinforces the display of appropriate behavior that serves the same function as the original target, challenging behavior.

Functional assessment data have been used successfully to design effective interventions for preschoolers with ADHD (Boyajian et al., 2001). Figure 1.1 displays data from a preschool-based functional (experimental) analysis for a 3-year-old child with ADHD (Jason) who participated in a study conducted by Boyajian et al. (2001). These data indicate that Jason's noncompliant, aggressive behavior was maintained by escape from task demands (i.e., the highest frequency of this behavior occurred during demand conditions). A brief test of contingency reversal (i.e., escape from demands presented following an alternative appropriate behavior, in this case making a request for a break, and withheld following noncompliant, aggressive behavior) showed increases in task engagement and decreases in noncompliance relative to baseline conditions (see Figure 1.2). Thus, intervention design is based on very specific data regarding the function of behavior and likelihood that a function-based intervention will be successful.

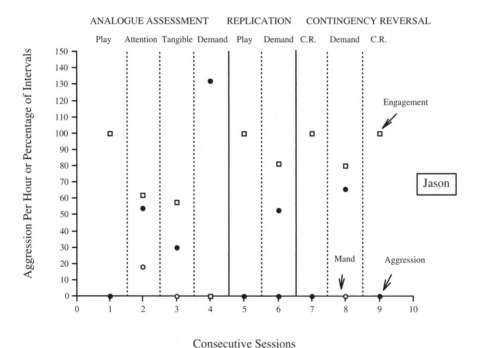

*Figure 1.1.* Level of aggression, requests (mands), and percentage of engagement across conditions in the analogue assessment, replication, and contingency reversal (C. R.) phases for Jason. From "The Use of Classroom-Based Brief Functional Analyses With Preschoolers at-Risk for Attention Deficit Hyperactivity Disorder," by A. E. Boyajian, G. J. DuPaul, M. W. Handler, T. L. Eckert, & K. E. McGoey, 2001, *School Psychology Review, 30,* p. 287. Copyright 2001 by the National Association of School Psychologists, Bethesda, MD. Reprinted with permission of the publisher. www.nasponline.org

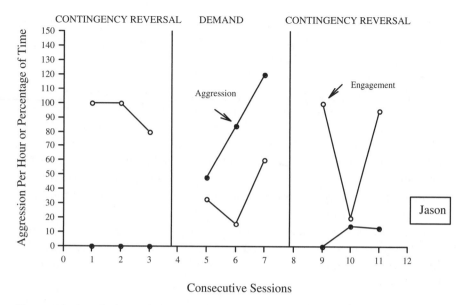

*Figure 1.2.* Level of aggression, requests, and percentage of engagement in the contingency reversal (i.e., intervention) and baseline (demand) phases for Jason. From "The Use of Classroom-Based Brief Functional Analyses With Preschoolers At-Risk for Attention Deficit Hyperactivity Disorder," by A. E. Boyajian, G. J. DuPaul, M. W. Handler, T. L. Eckert, & K. E. McGoey, 2001, *School Psychology Review, 30,* p. 290. Copyright 2001 by the National Association of School Psychologists, Bethesda, MD. Reprinted with permission of the publisher. www.nasponline.org

## ONGOING COLLECTION OF ASSESSMENT DATA

Once intervention strategies are implemented, assessment data should be collected periodically to document whether treatment is successful. For example, direct observations of target behavior(s) can be conducted before and after intervention to document treatment-induced changes in level, trend, and intercept. Another option would be to collect teacher and parent ratings of ADHD symptoms (using narrowband rating scales) both before and after intervention. It also is important to identify whether treatment reduces academic and social impairments that are associated with ADHD symptoms by using rating scales, direct observations, or direct measures of functioning. Stated differently, treatment efficacy is based not solely on reduction of ADHD-related behaviors but also on clinically significant improvements in functioning at home and school. If data indicate no improvement or only partial improvement, then changes to intervention should be considered, selected, implemented, and evaluated in an iterative fashion.

In our research on early intervention, we collect data regarding symptom change as well as academic, behavioral, and social functioning every

6 months to monitor functional trajectories over time. This period between assessments allows for treatment effects to occur and precludes concerns regarding "practice" effects biasing repeated measurements using the same instrument. Further, it is important to collect data that involve multiple respondents (i.e., parents and teachers) and varied modes of measurement (e.g., rating scales, direct observations) so that the limitations of any one measure or respondent are counterbalanced by the strengths of other measures or respondents. For example, rating scale data may reflect, in part, the biased perceptions of the respondent and can be balanced by direct observations conducted by a neutral observer who presumably does not share similar biases. Finally, ongoing measurement of treatment response should take advantage of existing measures designed to document change over time. Curriculum-based assessment of early reading and math skills are preferred over standardized, norm-referenced indices (e.g., Woodcock–Johnson Test of Educational Achievement) because of their relative brevity and use of alternate forms.

## CONCLUSIONS

ADHD is a disorder that typically begins early in life and is associated with chronic academic or social impairment (or both). It is important to identify young children who may meet diagnostic criteria for this disorder as early as possible so that effective interventions can be implemented in home, preschool, and day care settings. In this chapter, we reviewed psychometrically sound methods to screen for and comprehensively assess ADHD symptoms and associated impairments in young children. A comprehensive assessment of ADHD and related disruptive behavior disorders requires multiple measures obtained across home, preschool, and day care settings using information from multiple respondents (parents, teachers, and care providers). There are four core methods used to assess behavior: structured interviews, standardized rating scales, direct observations of behavior, and, in rare cases, direct measures of attention and hyperactivity–impulsivity. Although far from perfect, the *DSM–IV–TR* diagnostic criteria are the best available standards to use for interpreting assessment data to make diagnostic decisions. We have emphasized that assessment does not end with a diagnostic decision but must be used to select, design, and evaluate interventions, as described in subsequent chapters. Diagnostic assessment of young children is challenging given a variety of developmental issues; however, if psychometrically sound measures are used and prudent diagnostic decisions are made, then children will be in position to receive effective early intervention that may ameliorate or prevent chronic academic and social difficulties.

# 2

# OVERVIEW OF AN EARLY INTERVENTION MODEL

Intervention for problematic behavior in preschool children has advanced considerably in the past 2 decades. One advance is the development of models of intervention to guide practitioners and interventionists. A recent model that is proving highly effective is intervention introduced in a tiered fashion, whereby less intrusive approaches are first implemented, with more intrusive strategies used only for nonresponders (e.g., Müller, 2007; Sugai & Horner, 2002). There are many advantages to tiered intervention. One benefit is that all children receive support of some sort, which is designed both to prevent problem behaviors from emerging and to diminish those already present. Also, many children respond to interventions that are relatively less labor-intensive to implement, with much smaller numbers of children requiring more intensive intervention. This allows resources to be allocated in a cost-efficient manner.

Another advance in the area of problem behavior is the increased understanding of the importance of early intervention. Intervention efforts are likely to be much less intensive when they are introduced when problems first emerge, before they are entrenched in a child's repertoire. Further, early intervention can prevent or decrease the unfavorable events that typically follow recurrent problem behavior, such as social rejection and academic failure.

Finally, there is an increasing consensus that treatment is most effective when it can be delivered across settings. This is particularly important for children with or at risk for attention-deficit/hyperactivity disorder (ADHD), who, by nature of the disorder, exhibit problems across multiple environments. When children experience the same type of structured environments with clear expectations, relevant supports, and consistent responses from all care providers, behavior will improve most rapidly and dramatically.

In this chapter, we describe a model of intervention based on the aforementioned principles. The model consists of a tiered, multisetting approach designed for young children with or at risk for ADHD. We begin by offering a brief history and rationale for the model. Then we describe adaptations of the model for preschool and day care environments and for home settings. Finally, we discuss ways that interventionists, such as clinical child psychologists, school psychologists, and behavior specialists, can function as effective consultants and collaborators when working with teachers, staff, and family members.

## DESCRIPTION OF EARLY INTERVENTION MODEL

Children with ADHD, perhaps more than any other disability or disorder, exhibit a range of behavior problems with respect to both topography and intensity. Hence, the most parsimonious intervention approach involves a tiered model, which is designed to provide a continuum of supports depending on child need (Horner, Sugai, Todd, & Lewis-Palmer, 2006). This model introduces Tier 1, or *universal intervention*, with a given population of individuals. Interventions within this tier are evidence-based strategies that are generally effective with large numbers of individuals within the population. Tier 2, or *secondary intervention*, is used only with individuals who are not responsive to intervention at the universal level. Intervention at this tier is usually delivered in a small-group format and involves specialized intervention or instruction. Finally, Tier 3, or *tertiary intervention*, is reserved for a small percentage of the population who exhibit intensive and intransigent behavior problems that are not responsive to Tier 2 secondary interventions. Tertiary intervention is individualized and generally derived from assessment information.

This model of prevention and intervention is now commonly used in schools throughout the United States in the form of schoolwide positive behavior support (SWPBS; Sugai & Horner, 2002) and response to intervention (RtI; Fuchs & Fuchs, 2006). In these two prominent models, Tier 1, universal intervention, is used with a school's entire student body. In the case of SWPBS, Tier 1 involves establishing schoolwide behavioral expectations, instructing students on those expectations, and providing rewards for following expectations and consistent consequences for failing to adhere to expectations. Tier 1 RtI consists of implementing evidence-based academic programs, such as a research-supported reading curriculum, with all students. Tier 2 provides more intensive, targeted interventions, such as social skills instruction in the case of SWPBS or small-group academic practice in RtI models. Finally, Tier 3 involves individualized intervention to address more serious behavior or academic problems. For example, Tier 3 SWPBS intervention usually includes an individualized intervention plan derived from a functional behavioral assessment (Kern, Hilt-Panahon, & Sokol, 2009). An example of a Tier 3 academic intervention in an RtI model is instruction in a remedial reading program (e.g., Fuchs & Fuchs, 2006).

A tiered model is particularly applicable for young children with or at risk for ADHD for several reasons. First, our prior research demonstrated that many behavior problems characteristic of young children with ADHD can be successfully eliminated with Tier 1 approaches (Kern et al., 2007). This renders the approach highly cost-effective because intervention at this level requires relatively less time and effort, compared with Tier 2 or 3 interventions. In addition, although particularly beneficial to children with ADHD, Tier 1 approaches can be advantageous to all children in preschool, day care, or home settings (e.g., Sokol, Kern, Arbolino, Thomas, & DuPaul, 2009). For instance, structure and developmentally appropriate practices facilitate the growth and development of all young children (Bredekamp & Copple, 1996). Further, because resources available through preschools or the community are generally limited, the available services can be effectively and cost-efficiently apportioned to address the needs of all children, expending intensive resources only when indicated. This is particularly important given the high incidence of ADHD and the potentially great costs associated with this disorder over the life span (Pelham, Foster, & Robb, 2007).

## EVALUATING RESPONSIVENESS TO INTERVENTION

A tiered approach to intervention is designed to deliver effective practices to all children, with the level of support determined by child need. An important part of the model is developing a procedure to establish the level of support that each child will receive. SWPBS models typically use office disciplinary referrals to determine the need for more intensive intervention. That is, after Tier 1 intervention has been introduced, students who continue to experience a high rate of office referrals are considered to be nonresponders in need of Tier 2 or 3 intervention. Office disciplinary referrals are a reasonable metric because they generally are administered for serious behavioral infractions (e.g., aggression, disrespect), rather than for minor problems that routinely occur in classrooms (e.g., off task, talking out of turn). In fact, SWPBS systems include training so that school staff members consistently administer office referrals for predetermined behavioral infractions. When used in this way, referrals typically identify students with behavior problems that genuinely warrant additional intervention. In addition, office disciplinary referrals do not require extensive staff effort, as do other forms of behavior monitoring, such as direct observation.

In schools with RtI models, some type of ongoing academic progress monitoring is used to determine the appropriate level of intervention. For example, in the case of reading intervention, the number of words read correctly per minute is the most common form of analysis. Brief, 3-minute probes are administered regularly to gauge student progress, and standardized data are available to determine where students stand with respect to their same-age peers. Students who are not achieving as expected move through tiers to receive more intensive intervention.

Determining responsiveness to intervention for young children with ADHD is not as straightforward as SWPBS and RtI procedures. One reason is that it is not possible to use a single metric to measure intervention need because behavior problems vary widely in topography, ranging from inattention to aggression and defiance. In addition, behavior problems tend to be fairly intensive from the start. For instance, as we noted earlier, most preschool-age children exhibit high rates of activity; hence, to be labeled with ADHD requires activity levels far exceeding the norm. Also, developmental differences can vary widely when children are very young. Those who have had little exposure to preacademic activities or who are second-language learners may have brief attention spans when they first enter a preschool and experience these new concepts. Children with extended prior experience with letters, numbers, and books often sustain their attention to such activities for longer periods of time. Finally, adults have different expectations with respect to both behavior and preacademic skills. For example, some teachers have high tolerance levels when it comes to child activity level and noise. This can make it difficult to determine whether more intensive intervention is necessary.

Because of the complexities involved in determining intervention responsiveness, we recommend several guidelines. First, behavior targeted for change should be individually determined. That is, given the range of problems that children with ADHD exhibit, attempting to identify a single behavior and related metric, as in SWPBS or RtI, is not adequately encompassing. For these reasons, it is best to prioritize behavior problems individually, with the first priority given to those that are likely to be dangerous to the child or others (Janney & Snell, 2000).

A second guideline when evaluating response to intervention is to consider the initial frequency or intensity of problem behavior and the progress that follows. Because a label of ADHD implies behavior problems far exceeding the norm, improvements in behavior should be evaluated, rather than considering only pure frequency or intensity. For example, when a child is seldom on task, engagement throughout half of an activity may represent a substantial improvement, even though it may still be far lower than typical peer engagement. In this situation, the child might be considered highly responsive to intervention, as long as engagement continues to move in this desired direction.

Finally, as each intervention tier is introduced, a sufficient amount of time should be allocated for the intervention to have an effect. This is particularly true because when new interventions are introduced, behavior sometimes worsens before it improves. For example, when a child is accustomed to staying up past her bedtime, she may initially engage in more intensive behavior problems when the parents attempt to follow through with bedtime. Similarly, when classroom routines are initially implemented, it may take time for children to become familiar with the new expectations, and they may be resistant to the loss of social time.

For the general population of school-age students, tiered approaches to intervention appear to have a fairly predictable configuration with respect to intervention responsiveness. Numerous studies have examined the way that a given school's population falls with respect to intervention tiers. In the case of both SWPBS and RtI, the majority of students (approximately 80%) will be responsive to Tier 1 universal intervention. Approximately 15% of the students in a given school will succeed at Tier 2, secondary intervention. The remaining approximately 5% of students will require intensive behavioral or academic supports.

Because of the intensity of behavior problems exhibited by the population of young children with or at risk for ADHD, larger numbers require Tiers 2 and 3 interventions. Although data are limited, our preliminary research suggests that approximately 40% of children will be responsive to Tier 1 intervention (Kern et al., 2007). For another approximately 40%, Tier 2 intervention is sufficient to result in acceptable behavioral improvements. The remaining roughly 20% of children will require intensive Tier 3 intervention. Even given the lower levels of responsiveness compared with schoolwide interventions, the model still represents a cost- and labor-efficient approach. In addition, the model allows for a good match between need and intervention type.

In the case of severe behavior problems, it may be necessary to implement intensive intervention (Tier 2 or 3) immediately. Several factors should be considered when considering the need to implement an intensive intervention quickly. First, the severity of symptoms should be evaluated. If problem behavior is resulting in injury to the child (self-injury) or others (aggression), or if it is causing serious social problems, intensive intervention should be introduced immediately. Second, the severity of impairment associated with behavior problems should be determined. For instance, if the severity of inattention interferes with learning basic preacademic skills, intensive intervention is usually warranted. Third, the likelihood of earlier tiers resulting in a reduction in problem behavior should be considered. For example, in preschool settings where a child is unable to follow any teacher rules or routines, Tier 1 intervention (establishing classwide expectations) is unlikely to reduce problem behaviors. In this case, Tier 2 or 3 intervention should be introduced immediately. It should also be noted that more intensive interventions (e.g., functional behavioral assessment–based intervention) can be implemented simultaneously with Tier 1 intervention (e.g., parent education, classwide expectations).

## DEVELOPING A COMPREHENSIVE APPROACH TO INTERVENTION

Children with ADHD experience a variety of difficulties that seldom occur in isolation (see Introduction and Chapter 1, this volume). Evident at a young age, these problems may include (a) defiant and aggressive behavior (Loeber, Green, Keenan, & Lahey, 1995; Offord, Boyle, & Racine, 1991), (b) difficulties with peer interactions and relationships (e.g., Barkley, 2006), (c) absence of preacademic readiness skills (Campbell et al., 1986; McGee et al., 1991), and (d) a high rate of accidental physical injuries (Lahey et al., 1998, 2004; Mitchell, Aman, Turbott, & Manku, 1987; Szatmari, Offord, & Boyle, 1989). Although not all children with ADHD will display all of these problems, because they frequently coexist, it is important to evaluate the presence of each and determine the need for intervention (e.g., Barkley, 2006). Further, these particular problems can have a substantial impact on child functioning and future prognosis. For instance, difficulties interacting with peers at an early age can lead to later problems making and maintaining friends, an important variable contributing to later quality of life (Milich, Landau, Kilby, & Whitten, 1982; S. M. R. Watson & Keith, 2002; Wehmeyer & Schalock, 2001). Similarly, children who have deficits in preacademic skills are more likely to experience later academic difficulties (Gersten & Jordan, 2005; Good, Simmons, & Smith, 1998; Juel, 1988). A comprehensive intervention plan will address all of the aforementioned problems that a given child exhibits.

In addition to addressing each problem area, intervention should be delivered in every environment where problems are present or likely to be present. As defined by the *Diagnostic and Statistical Manual of Mental Disorders* (4th ed., text revision; *DSM–IV–TR*; American Psychiatric Association, 2000), to receive a diagnosis of ADHD, symptoms must be present across more than a single setting (see Chapter 1, this volume). It light of this, it is important to note that a great deal of intervention research has demonstrated that the effects of intervention implemented in one setting do not necessarily generalize to other settings (e.g., Chandler, 1992; Stokes, 1992). To ensure that desirable behavior is exhibited across environments, interventions must be learned and practiced in each setting in which children typically spend time. Preschool-age children generally spend the majority of their time in home and preschool or day care settings. Thus, intervention delivered in these two settings usually covers most of a child's day. Further, interventionists will be those individuals (parents and care providers, preschool and day care teachers and staff) who interact with the child most frequently and are positioned to deliver intervention most frequently. When multisetting intervention is consistently delivered by the primary care providers in those settings, intervention effects are likely to be most pervasive across environments.

## OVERVIEW OF HOME-BASED TIERED MODEL

To date, there is limited research evaluating a tiered model of support in home settings for young children with ADHD. There is, however, a strong rationale for its use. First, home-based intervention poses unique challenges (see Exhibit 2.1), particularly because it is often difficult to gain access to home environments, and even when access is obtained, the provision of home-based services is costly. Thus, the Tier 1 intervention we have identified (parent education) is particularly advantageous because it can be delivered outside of the home setting, avoiding the problem with accessibility and expenditure for home visits. In addition, the Tier 1 intervention we have tested (e.g., Kern et al., 2007) can be delivered in a group format, reducing the cost per individual family. Finally, our preliminary research indicates that Tier 1 intervention will result in significant reductions in behavior problems for a large percentage of young children with symptoms of ADHD, making it an effective initial approach to intervention.

Tier 1 home-based intervention consists of parent education focused on addressing the major questions parents have concerning their child and arming them with intervention strategies to reduce behavior problems, increase appropriate and desirable behavior, prevent accidental injuries, and introduce preacademic skills. Parent education begins with an overview of symptoms of

## EXHIBIT 2.1
### Challenges to Implementation of Interventions

*Issue: We do not have the resources in our preschool to implement Tier 3, individualized interventions.*

Potential Solution: Tier 3 interventions are labor-intensive. However, most educators spend a great deal of time addressing problem behaviors. Often they are unaware of the numerous minutes spent throughout the day correcting children's problem behavior. A tiered approach to intervention can prevent most problem behaviors and reduces the overall need for more intensive, Tier 2 and 3, interventions. In general, less time is spent with behavior management overall when a tiered approach is used.

*Issue: The teachers in our preschool expect to see immediate change when behavior interventions are implemented and are prone to give up when behavior problems continue.*

Potential Solution: When preschool teachers develop and implement interventions, it is reasonable to have high expectations for success. It is equally important to keep in mind that children need to learn new ways of behavior, which may not come immediately. For this reason, it is important to collect data and celebrate progress in the form of small improvements, rather than expecting immediate elimination of problem behavior.

*Issue: Terrance engages in constant problem behaviors at preschool, but his parents claim he does not have problems at home and refuse to believe he is so troublesome at preschool.*

Potential Solution: It is important to understand that expectations at preschool may be very different from those at home. For example, at preschool, children are expected to engage in preacademic learning activities. This requires attending to teacher instruction for sustained periods of time (e.g., 10–15 minutes), which may not be required at home. Also, children are required to interact socially with their peers in an appropriate manner, such as sharing toys and jointly participating in activities. Children may not be accustomed to this type of social requirement, particular those without siblings. Finally, parent tolerance for problem behavior varies widely. Some parents do not mind extremely active or boisterous children. Thus, it is important to help parents understand what is required at school and to be specific about the types of behaviors that are problematic.

ADHD, along with the typical sequelae of the disorder and the importance of early intervention. This is followed by basic behavioral intervention strategies urging parents and care providers to reward appropriate child behavior, ignore minor inappropriate behavior, and follow through with instructions and expectations. In addition, parents learn techniques to prevent universal problems, such as difficulties making the transition from one activity to another and, in the case of families with multiple children, balancing their attention across children. Also, to decrease accidental injuries, home safety is covered, including safety-proofing the home and monitoring children. Finally, because young children with ADHD tend to lag behind their peers in basic math and prereading skills, parents are provided an array of activities to improve their child's early literacy and numeracy skills and to prepare him or her for entry into kindergarten.

During the parent education sessions, a number of instructional techniques are used to enhance the likelihood that parents and care providers will fully understand the rationale and procedures for implementing intervention strategies (Codding, Feinberg, Dunn, & Pace, 2005; Mortenson & Witt, 1998; Noell, Witt, Gilbertson, Ranier, & Freeland, 1997). First, the technique is described, along with an explanation of how and why it is effective. In addition, video clips and modeling by the facilitator allow parents to observe the strategy being implemented. This is followed by role play to make sure the parents are able to implement each step of the strategy as designed and have practice doing so. Finally, time is allotted for questions. During the following session, parents share successes and challenges implementing the intervention and brainstorm ways to enhance implementation.

Parents are convened into groups of approximately 10 to 12 families and proceed through the sessions as a cohort. This grouping is advantageous for several reasons. First, as previously noted, providing intervention simultaneously to multiple parents is cost-efficient. In addition, parents report feeling at ease and having a sense of support in the presence of other families experiencing similar challenges with their children. Finally, parents are able to share tips about when and how they implemented the interventions.

Given the importance of parent education sessions, strategies should be implemented to increase the likelihood of attendance. A number of techniques have been shown to increase session attendance (e.g., Robinson, Dennison, Wayman, Pronovost, & Needham, 2007). First, sessions should be scheduled at a time that is most convenient for the parents in a given cohort. Because most parents work, this usually means evenings or weekends. In addition, providing cab or bus fare or arranging for car pools avoids transportation barriers. Offering child care for siblings and providing food also enhance attendance. Finally, an additional tangible incentive can improve attendance. We designed a lottery system in which parents at each session complete a lottery card. One card is randomly drawn periodically throughout the education course, and the family selected receives a $25 gift certificate.

For children who continue to exhibit problem behavior following Tier 1 intervention, Tier 2 involves home-based coaching in the strategies taught during parent education. For some parents, the instruction and practice provided during parent education sessions are not sufficient for them to implement the techniques consistently. Sometimes this happens because parents have entrenched patterns of interacting with their children or responding to problem behavior that are difficult for them to change. Other times children exhibit unique problems, or they exhibit problems in unusual situations, requiring slight modifications of the strategies.

During individual coaching sessions, each technique that was taught in the parent education sessions is reviewed. Coaching sessions are intentionally scheduled during times when the child is likely to engage in problem behaviors. The home-based consultant observes the parent implementing each step of the strategy, providing feedback on implementation accuracy and additional instruction as needed. In addition, the consultant may adjust the strategy to accommodate unique child behaviors or situations. For example, if a parent is able to provide reinforcement for appropriate behavior when the target child is alone with the parent but is unable to do so when siblings are present, additional strategies may be designed, such as a timer that sounds periodically to remind the parent to attend to the target child.

As noted earlier, Tier 3 intervention is introduced for the relatively small number of children that do not respond to Tier 2 intervention. Similar to Tier 3 intervention in the preschool setting, an individualized support plan is developed on the basis of a functional assessment. In the home, the parents or care providers are taught to collect data indicating what problem behavior occurred, what preceded the problem behavior, and how they responded to the problem. Parent data are supplemented by direct observation data collected by the consultant. In addition, functional analyses can be conducted to provide specificity on events that precede and reinforce problem behavior. Specifically, situations are arranged to evaluate whether commonly known functions account for problem behavior. These testable functions for problem behavior include obtaining attention, escaping tasks or demands, and obtaining preferred items or activities.

After the functional assessment has been completed, interventions are developed with components identical to preschool assessment-based interventions. That is, the environment can be modified to prevent problems, alternative skills can be taught to the child, and ways of responding to problem behavior can be identified so that it is not reinforced.

## OVERVIEW OF INTERVENTION MODEL
## FOR PRESCHOOL AND DAY CARE SETTINGS

There is a strong rationale, accompanied by growing empirical support, for a tiered approach to intervention in preschool and day care settings (e.g., Fox, Dunlap, Hemmeter, Joseph, & Strain, 2003). First, although young children with characteristics of ADHD may need specialized and individualized supports to reduce their behavior problems and ensure that they are learning, many will be responsive to less intensive classroom interventions. As we noted earlier, this makes intervention cost- and labor-efficient. In addition, having fundamental classwide interventions and practices in place creates a positive classroom environment, teaches appropriate behaviors rather than focusing on and punishing problem behaviors, and ensures that learning opportunities are optimized for all children. Further, classwide interventions set the stage for introducing more intensive interventions, as well as determining whether they are needed. Specifically, it is difficult to introduce individualized interventions in a classroom that is chaotic or one in which practices are not appropriate. For example, when circle time in a preschool lasts a full hour, this exceeds the attention span of almost all 3- to 5-year-old children. Hence, developing an intervention for the child with ADHD symptoms would be both difficult and contraindicated. When circle time is of an appropriate duration, matched to the length of time most preschool age students should be able to sustain their attention, then it is easy to identify those students who need additional intervention or support. Also, when solid classwide practices are in place, intervention is more likely to be effective because the majority of the class should be attending. Good role models surround the child, children are receiving reinforcement for attending, and there is no competition to change the behavior of a single student amid an entire classroom of children with similar difficulties.

Tier 1 intervention for preschool day care settings involves all individuals, as do SWPBS and RtI. Rather than intervention at the schoolwide level, in this setting, universal intervention usually targets the classroom. In large programs with multiple preschool classrooms, classwide intervention can be consistent across classrooms. Classwide intervention is designed to improve practices for all children in a classroom. For example, classroom rules or expectations are developed so that all children learn what is expected of their behavior. This is accompanied by systems of reinforcement so that children are rewarded for engaging in appropriate behavior and recognize that there are clear and consistent consequences when they do not follow expectations. In addition, Tier 1 intervention involves structuring activities throughout the school day so that they are developmentally appropriate or matched to the developmental level of preschool-age children.

Tier 2 offers more intensive support, specifically targeting nonresponders. For example, if a few children continue to engage in problem behavior during play time, small-group social skills instruction may be provided. Instruction may focus on a particular problem, such as sharing or turn taking.

Intervention at Tier 3 is individualized and linked to the assessment results. This involves conducting a functional assessment to identify the exact nature of problem behavior and determine what events precede and follow problem behavior. The assessment information allows interventions to be developed that restructure the environment, provide necessary skill instruction, and identify adult responses that are unlikely to reinforce child behavior. This assessment-based and individualized approach to intervention is efficient for ongoing problem behavior because, rather than randomly selecting an intervention from the large host of options, assessment information suggests classes of interventions that are likely to be effective.

## COLLABORATING AND CONSULTING

Consultation has taken a turn in recent years, with a current emphasis on collaboration (Erchul & Martens, 2010). Consultants, such as school psychologists, behavior specialists, and other individuals who facilitate intervention for children with problem behavior, have a certain skill and knowledge set. At the same time, family members and preschool staff and day care providers also have unique knowledge of and experiences with the target child. For instance, family members have generally been with their child since birth, spend numerous hours each day with their child, and have a vested interest in his or her long-term outcomes. In this way, they bring special understanding and interests. These different forms of knowledge are all valuable for building a support plan. Hence, intervention can best be derived through partnership.

In addition to the specialized knowledge of family members and professional staff, each setting in which intervention will be implemented presents distinctive environmental characteristics that must be taken into account when designing intervention. For example, if a preschool classroom is populated with 25 children, providing ongoing attention to any individual child can be arduous. Family situations also differ widely in the number of people in the household, parenting skills and attitudes, parental stress level, and harmony or discord among family members. These variables can affect a parent's willingness and ability to implement intervention procedures. Thus, collaboration is critical to ensure that support plans offer a good ecological fit. In other words, the plan must be consistent with the values of those implementing it, and they should be able to carry it out in typical day-to-day settings. Certain practices can enhance and facilitate the collaboration process.

An important first step is to fully understand the priorities of the preschool or day care staff and families with respect to intervention (Fleming & Monda-Amaya, 2001; Straka & Bricker, 1996). When those collaborating do not agree on behaviors that need to be reduced or skills that should be improved, a support plan is sure to fail. Hence, all parties should first agree on intervention goals. When doing so, it is important to keep in mind that individuals have different expectations for the future and varying degrees of tolerance for particular types of problem behaviors. Janney and Snell (2000) offered a useful heuristic for prioritizing behavior problems. One class of behavior, considered *distracting,* is that which deviates from expected norms (e.g., inappropriate interactions, hand flapping) but does not substantially interfere with learning or typical activities. Distracting behaviors should be considered the lowest intervention priority. Behaviors in another category, *disruptive* (e.g., refusing to complete assignments, yelling), do not pose immediate danger to the student or others but interfere with learning and the environment. These should be the next priority for intervention. Finally, *destructive* behaviors are harmful or threaten the safety of the student or others (e.g., aggression, property destruction, bringing weapons to school, self-harm) and are the first priority for intervention.

In addition to coming to consensus about the behaviors in need of change, it is important that preschool staff and family members understand the intervention process. Specifically, it is critical to fully recognize the link between environmental events and behavior. This is particularly true when working with children with ADHD because it is often assumed that behavior such as overactivity is biologically determined and cannot be controlled. Those working with children with ADHD must understand that there is a relationship between the environment and occurrences of problem behavior. Regardless of the cause of problem behavior, environmental changes can reduce it (e.g., Dunlap, Harrower, & Fox, 2005). Preschool or day care staff and family members need to realize that *their* behavior must change for the child's behavior to change.

Finally, it is important to address conflicts systematically, should they arise. Developing a strategy for conflict resolution is especially important given that intervention will be implemented over a substantial period of time (e.g., DuPaul & Stoner, 2003). A number of articles, books, and research studies describe and evaluate effective strategies for problem solving (e.g., Isaksen, Treffinger, & Dorval, 2000; McNamara, Dennis, & Carte, 2008; Snell & Janney, 2000). The research spans diverse disciplines but, for the most part, depicts analogous steps. Further, most research suggests that the particular strategy used is not as important as approaching the problem in a systematic manner (LaFasto & Larson, 2001).

## PROBLEM SOLVING

Regardless of a practitioner's skill and experience with collaboration, problems are bound to arise from time to time. It is important to have a problem-solving process in place in these situations. This section describes a generic five-step problem-solving framework.

The first step is to identify the problem. When a problem arises, those involved should come to consensus about the exact issue that needs to be resolved. At times, particularly when family members or preschool or day care staff feel overwhelmed with a child's problem behavior, there may seem to be multiple problems. In these situations, one issue should be addressed at a time, with the single, most important addressed first. The problem definition should focus on identifying a solution rather than simply acknowledging the problem. For example, the statement "The preschool refuses to implement the intervention" is not solution focused. An alternative and solution-focused way to state the problem is, "We need to determine what supports and training are needed for the preschool to be able to implement the intervention."

After the problem is identified, the next step is to brainstorm possible solutions. *Brainstorming* is a collaborative process that allows all parties involved to generate potential solutions. There are a number of specific brainstorming techniques. For example, during *group passing*, each individual writes an idea on a piece of paper then passes it to another group member to add to the thought. Another method is *team idea mapping*, in which each individual brainstorms independently and then ideas are combined onto a large map. During brainstorming, the goal is to come up with as many solutions as possible. Creative and unusual solutions are welcome and should not be evaluated or criticized at this stage.

Following brainstorming, the potential solutions are analyzed during the third step. Before evaluating potential solutions, it is sometimes helpful to generate a list of criteria for evaluating each idea (Janney & Snell, 2000). For example, when considering how to improve intervention implementation in a preschool setting, it may be important to consider whether the teacher can implement the intervention, how much the child's behavior is likely to improve, and whether the intervention is likely to be stigmatizing. Each solution is analyzed, narrowing ideas to those that are likely to work best. Sometimes ideas can be combined to form a better solution than a single idea offers.

The fourth step is to select a solution. Ideally, this is accomplished through consensus. At times, however, there may be more than one acceptable solution, or individuals may differ on what they believe is the best solution. In these cases, a solution can be identified through vote or compromise. It also is important to keep in mind that one solution can be tried first, with the agreement that if the problem is not resolved successfully, another will be tried.

The final step is to develop a plan for implementing the solution. Because solutions are often just ideas, they need to be accompanied by specific steps and timelines for implementation. In addition, evaluation criteria can be established to determine whether the solution has worked.

# CONCLUSIONS

The newest advance in the area of intervention for problem behavior is a tiered model of support in which all children receive universal support, and intervention intensity increases only when children do not respond to less intensive intervention. A tiered approach focuses on prevention and is largely instructive. This approach is cost-efficient and appears to be particularly valuable and effective if implemented when children are very young. A tiered model is applicable in both home and preschool or day care settings, which is important for children with ADHD, who exhibit symptoms of the disorder in multiple settings. Tiered intervention can be organized and arranged by clinical child psychologists, school psychologists, behavior specialists, special education teachers, and other practitioners through a collaborative consultative model. When important steps are implemented, such as identifying a child behavior to target for intervention and developing a strategy for addressing problems, practitioners and families can work together productively and successfully.

# 3

# HOME-BASED BEHAVIORAL INTERVENTION STRATEGIES

Among very young children, the vast majority of interpersonal contact occurs with the child's parents. Even when children attend day care, they still spend significant amounts of time with their parents in the morning and evening hours and on weekends. During these early years, parent–child interactions play a significant role in child development (Levenstein, 1992). Parents of children with attention-deficit/hyperactivity disorder (ADHD), however, report feeling unprepared to address the challenges their children exhibit (e.g., Keown & Woodward, 2002; Sobol, Ashbourne, Earn, & Cunningham, 1989). In fact, research indicates that interactions between parents and their child with ADHD may be different from their interactions with their other children (e.g., C. E. Cunningham & Barkley, 1979). Patterson (1982) posited that coercive interactions, which occur during the toddler and preschool years, exacerbate behavior problems and can lead to the later development of conduct problems and antisocial behavior. Hence, home-based intervention is critical.

Home-based early intervention has distinct advantages. First, given that parents spend significant amounts of time with their children, implementation of effective behavioral strategies can be pervasive. Ongoing intervention implementation by family members throughout the day and across multiple settings (e.g., the home, community, homes of relatives and friends) increases the likelihood of rapid improvements in child behavior. Also, early intervention is more successful than later intervention because children have had limited opportunities to practice problem behaviors, and adult interaction style may be more malleable (J. B. Reid & Eddy, 1997). Further, parents play a significant role in shaping the behavior of their children at a young age, a role that diminishes over time as peers and outside environmental variables become more salient (Patterson, Reid, & Dishion, 1992). Perhaps most important, in the absence of early home-based intervention, behavior problems are likely to persist and worsen, frequently leading to more serious problems, such as conduct disorder (Lahey & Loeber, 1997).

Home-based intervention has proved successful in reducing the symptoms of ADHD in young children (e.g., Kern et al., 2007). Parents, however, differ in their ability to implement intervention consistently for various reasons, such as parental stress, competing environmental demands in the home, and their attitude toward and tolerance for behavior problems (e.g., C. E. Cunningham, Bremner, & Boyle, 1995). Thus, some parents need more support than others. Also, child responsiveness to intervention differs greatly. Responsiveness to intervention is not always predictable a priori; however, symptom severity seems to play a role in the intensity of the intervention required to reduce behavior problems (Egger, Kondo, & Angold, 2006). For these reasons, a tiered model is well suited to early home-based intervention in that it allows different levels or intensities of intervention to be implemented as indicated. Children who are nonresponsive should move through the tiers to a more intensive intervention. Also, when problem behavior is severe, Tier 3 intervention can be introduced immediately (or simultaneously with other tiers).

In this chapter, we describe a home-based tiered intervention model for young children with or at risk for ADHD. Within each intervention tier, we detail specific intervention strategies and supports.

## OVERVIEW OF HOME-BASED INTERVENTION MODEL

The tiered model of support described in this chapter introduces increasingly intensive support strategies on the basis of child need. This makes early intervention both efficient and cost-effective. Tier 1 intervention consists of *group-based parent education*. Our prior research (Kern et al., 2007) suggests that close to 40% of children with early symptoms of ADHD will be responsive to the interventions implemented in Tier 1. For children who continue to engage in behavior problems following Tier 1 approaches, Tier 2 provides additional practice and support in the form of *home-based coaching*. At this tier, parents receive in-home support to adapt the behavioral strategies to address both their child's specific needs and variables in the home situation. Coaching is provided to assist parents to implement the strategies with integrity. For the relatively small group of children with problem behavior that persists following Tier 1 and Tier 2 interventions, Tier 3 is introduced. At Tier 3, an individualized intervention is developed that is based on information gathered through the process of functional behavioral assessment. Thus, *assessment-based intervention* involves development of a comprehensive and multicomponent support plan for the home and community settings. In the sections that follow, we describe home-based intervention at each tier. See Figure 3.1 for an illustration of the home-based intervention model.

## TIER 1: GROUP-BASED PARENT EDUCATION

Tier 1 of home-based intervention consists of small-group parent education sessions. The content presented during these structured sessions is an important starting point for all families, regardless of the severity of their

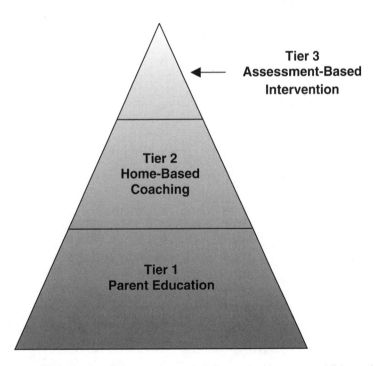

*Figure 3.1.* Illustration of tiered home-based intervention for young children with attention-deficit/hyperactivity disorder.

child's behavior problems, because it familiarizes parents with the diagnosis of ADHD and related issues, lays the foundation for understanding behavioral intervention, and helps parents learn techniques to address current and prevent future problems. With this foundation, parents find Tiers 2 and 3 interventions much easier to understand and implement, and consultation time is reduced at these later tiers.

Parents are grouped into cohorts for parent education in part because they report feeling relief when hearing that other families experience similar challenges with their children, and they benefit from accounts of other parents' success in implementing intervention strategies. In addition, it is cost-effective to provide sessions in a group format, and the discussion during sessions appears to enhance comprehension of the content. We recommend cohorts with approximately 10 families. Although a cohort can be smaller, larger ones pose difficulties when completing session activities. Further, it is difficult for the group leader to establish a close rapport with family members when cohorts are too large.

Because attendance can be a problem for parents with busy schedules and competing responsibilities, techniques suggested in the literature to enhance participation should be used. First, sessions should be scheduled at a time that is mutually convenient for all parents in a cohort, which generally is evenings or weekends. In addition, sessions should be centrally located near the homes of the participating families or at a familiar location where the parents regularly visit (e.g., child's school, local church). Also, when viable, the provision of free transportation and sibling child care makes it possible for those parents to participate who cannot drive or are unable to afford the child care needed for attendance. Finally, families enjoy snacks provided during the sessions. If parents are unable to attend a session, the materials can be sent to them for review either by e-mail or by post.

Our parent education program consists of ten 2-hour sessions. We hold sessions biweekly so that parents have sufficient time to practice the strategies taught in the sessions. Also, it often takes time for children to respond to the techniques after they are consistently implemented by parents. Thus, distributing sessions across 5 months allows adequate time to determine parent skill level at implementation and child responsiveness.

Sessions can be led by individuals with expertise and training in implementing behavioral interventions. In addition, experience consulting with families is important. Session leaders may include educators (e.g., teachers, school psychologists), behavior specialists, or community providers.

The first session, "Opening and Introduction to ADHD," introduces parents to one another and to the session leader(s). In addition, ADHD symptoms are described in detail, along with the potential negative sequelae if intervention is not sought. We begin the session with an enjoyable activity that helps parents get to know each other. For example, we have parents complete a short questionnaire about themselves and then compare answers with others in the group to find, for example, who has the most children, who has a pet, who is left-handed, who was born in the most distant state, who speaks the most languages, who likes sporting events, and so forth. In addition, confidentiality and respect are discussed. It is important that parents feel free to discuss their children's problems without derision and that they commit to keeping the discussion within the group. Subsequently, we discuss ADHD, including its history, prevalence rates, gender differences, subtypes, characteristics associated with subtypes, and common associated difficulties (i.e., problems with language, learning, behavior, social skills, emotional regulation). At the end of the session, we briefly discuss praise, including the content of praise statements and how to increase the ratio of praise to reprimands and provide parents with "101 Ways to Praise a Child" (e.g., http://www.character-kids.com). Increasing praise statements gives parents a technique they can use immediately, which can have a significant positive impact on child behavior. The immediate improvement parents often experience as a result of praise encourages them to return for future sessions.

Sessions 2 through 6 focus on instructing parents in critical behavior management strategies. We use the Community Parent Education (COPE) curriculum (C. E. Cunningham et al., 1998) for these sessions. The COPE is an empirically validated parent education program that has been used successfully in the past to reduce children's behavior problems. Further, the program is easily accessible, particularly with respect to affordability.

The focus of Session 2 is how to attend to and reward children's appropriate behavior. Parents learn to identify and rehearse strategies for showing interest in, encouraging, and rewarding their child's constructive play. In addition, the importance of cooperative interactions and prosocial child behaviors is stressed, particularly given that these are problematic areas for young children with ADHD. A variety of strategies are used to assist parents in providing high rates of rewards for appropriate behavior, improving interactions with their child, and reducing coercive exchanges. The COPE program contains videos that depict parents engaging in desirable and undesirable interactions with their children. Parents view the videos, then divide into subgroups to critique them and develop alternative responses. Next, the session leader models how parents can enhance interactions and provide their child praise during common activities at home. Parents then generate ideas about situations in their own homes in which they can engage in positive interactions and praise their children. Subsequently, parents practice engaging in productive interactions and providing praise via role play. Before ending the session, parents are provided homework activities for the next 2 weeks. In preparation for homework, they develop a specific plan for interacting positively with and praising their child (e.g., when, how), identify obstacles they might encounter, and generate solutions for overcoming obstacles.

Session 3 begins with a review of the previous homework assignment. Parents share their success with praise and positive interactions and brainstorm ways to address obstacles they encountered. Then, the topic of Session 3 turns to balanced attending and planned ignoring. The idea that children with ADHD can require a great deal of time and attention, taking time away from siblings, is discussed. Parents learn how to balance their time and attention among all children in their family, in addition to learning how to reward positive interactions between siblings. They also learn how attention can inadvertently reinforce common problem behaviors, such as whining, arguing, and engaging in tantrums. Parents learn to ignore these minor behavior problems. An additional focus is to work with parents to understand the ways that their own behavior may escalate their children's behavior. For example, children may engage in behaviors (e.g., saying "I hate you") to "get a rise" out of parents (i.e., get parental attention). Parents identify such behaviors, learning ways to disengage and counter their own thoughts that may intensify their anger. As in Session 2, parents view and critique videos of the appropriate and inappropriate use of balanced attending and planned ignoring. They generate alternative strategies for the inappropriate application of balanced attending depicted in the videos. In addition, the session leader models each of the strategies, followed by role play in parent dyads or triads to provide parents practice implementing the techniques. Finally, homework is again assigned, whereby parents identify concrete situations and goals for using the session's strategies at home. Parents are reminded not to expect immediate behavior change and are encouraged to generate ways to deal with extinction bursts that might occur when ignoring problem behavior. That is, because child problem behavior sometimes escalates when it no longer draws attention, parents propose ways they can deal with the escalation.

During Session 4, after parents review homework successes and generate solutions to obstacles, they learn about transitional warnings and when–then statements. The session leader describes how transitions, such as turning off the television, coming to the dinner table, and going to bed, can be difficult for children. Parents learn to give clear instructions, avoiding abrupt commands or pleading with children to comply. They are coached on ways to schedule and prepare their children for transitions, as well as how to follow through with instructions. In addition, parents learn how to apply the Premack principle (Premack, 1959) by scheduling pleasant activities following difficult or problematic tasks or activities and providing when–then statements (e.g., stating, "We can read a book as soon as you finish brushing your teeth"). As in Sessions 2 and 3, videos depict accurate and inaccurate applications of transitional warnings and when–then statements, facilitating discussion and alternative strategies. The session also includes the leader modeling the strategies and parent role-play in subgroups. In preparation for homework, parents establish specific goals about how and when they will use the strategies.

After homework review in the same format as Sessions 2 through 4, Session 5 covers the topics of point systems and time out from reinforcement. Point or token reward systems are encouraged, particularly for children who are not sufficiently responsive to the strategies previously taught for encouraging appropriate behavior and who need additional incentives. Parents learn how to design a simple incentive system, including selecting and defining target behaviors they will reward. Video clips facilitate discussion of common errors (e.g., intervals that are too long, behaviors that are vaguely defined, rewards that are not reinforcing) and how they can be corrected. Sample incentive systems are shared with parents, and time is allocated for parents to develop a system to use in their own home. Time out from reinforcement also is discussed during this session. Because time out can be overused, this topic is introduced after parents have had sufficient opportunity to learn about and practice providing reinforcement to their children, ignoring minor problem behaviors, issuing clear instructions and following through, and scheduling and transitioning successfully. Parents are taught when time out is likely to be effective and when it will not be effective. For example, parents learn to avoid time out when misbehavior involves avoiding task completion (e.g., going to bed, cleaning up toys) because the use of time out may actually serve to reinforce avoidant behavior. Parameters on the use of time out are reviewed (e.g., how long time out should be, how frequently it should be used). Videos are used to supplement instruction, followed by leader modeling and role play. Finally, homework involves planning when and how point systems and time out will be used in the home.

Following homework review, Session 6 focuses on planning ahead. During this session, parents learn how to plan for community activities and use effective management strategies across settings and in the presence of others. In addition, parents learn how to assist relatives, babysitters, and other individuals in implementing the strategies that are effective with their child. Videos show parents making errors such as publicly criticizing their child or forgetting to preplan for a home visitor. Parents discuss the errors, consequences of the errors, and alternatives to the errors. The session leader models ways to plan ahead, facilitated by scripts. For example, with a parent volunteering to play the role of a child, the leader informs the child that they are going to the grocery store, asks the child to describe some good things he could do at the store, then plans how the child can help with the shopping. When they arrive at the store, the leader (playing the parent) asks the child to remind her of how he is going to help at the store. The leader (as parent) then demonstrates how to prompt and praise the child. Parents role play other scenarios in small groups. Homework preparation involves identifying concrete goals by determining when and how planning ahead will be used. Homework is reviewed during the next session with the approach used in Sessions 2 through 5.

Session 7 focuses on safety, such as safety proofing the home and monitoring children (see Chapter 6). This session is important given the high rate of accidental injuries among children with ADHD. The Injury Prevention Program (TIPP; American Academy of Pediatrics, 1999a) was used to develop this session. Numerous types of injury prevention strategies are described in areas such as falls, bike safety, toy safety, choking, burns, gun safety, poisons, car safety, pedestrian safety, and water safety. Video clips are used to demonstrate injury prevention. Parents complete the TIPP safety survey (http://www. aap.org/family/tippmain.htm) and discuss answers to their surveys. Parents develop a homework plan to prevent injuries to their child at home by modifying their behavior (e.g., enhancing supervision) and the physical environment (e.g., rearranging furniture to prevent injuries, moving small objects that pose a choking hazard out of reach). At the following session, parents discuss changes they made and how they affected child behavior or may do so in the future.

Sessions 8 and 9 are designed to address the fact that children with ADHD lag behind their peers in prereading and early math skills (see Chapter 5). These sessions offer an overview of early skill development in reading and math concepts. In addition, parents are taught activities to improve their child's numeracy and literacy skills. For example, activities focus on blending sounds, blending syllables, segmenting syllables, letter–sound correspondence, rhyming, identifying numbers, naming numbers, and so forth. In addition, parents are provided activities obtained from the Ladders to Literacy curriculum (Notari-Syverson, O'Conner, & Vadasy, 1998). The activities from this curriculum can be embedded into ongoing routines and are excellent for parents who are busy. Similar activities are provided for parents to work with their children in development of numeracy skills.

The final session is designed to ensure that parents and their children are prepared for kindergarten. Child readiness skills are discussed, and parents are provided additional strategies to assist their child with the skills needed to succeed in kindergarten in a number of areas, such as self-help, self-control, and social interactions. In addition, parents learn about their rights with respect to school-based evaluation, services, and due process. Special education and accommodations are discussed, including Individualized Education Plans and 504 Plans. As part of this session, parents become familiar with the education and special education system, practice effective communication with educators, and learn ways to advocate effectively for their child.

After parent education sessions are completed, we assess whether children have been responsive to this tier of intervention. Responsiveness can be evaluated through direct observations conducted during home visits, parents' reports of successes and difficulties managing their child's behavior, or professionals' (e.g., social worker, teacher) recommendations regarding parent behavior management skills or reported and observed child difficulties. When evaluating responsiveness, we primarily consider improvements in child behavior. Our prior research indicates that when children show improvement within the first 6 months of intervention, those improvements are likely to continue (Kern et al., 2007). When improvements are not observed or are minimal, Tier 2 intervention is introduced. Also, as noted previously, the severity of a child's problem behaviors (e.g., frequent aggression, dangerous behavior) occasionally requires intensive intervention immediately, and Tier 2 or 3 interventions should not be delayed in such circumstances.

## TIER 2: HOME-BASED COACHING

For children who do not show adequate improvement after parent education, Tier 2 intervention, consisting of home-based coaching, is introduced. The intent of intervention at Tier 2 is to provide parents with additional coaching and practice implementing the interventions learned during parent education and to tailor the interventions to address individual home environments and parent needs. Generally, 10 sessions are conducted in the family's home, each lasting 2 hours. Parents are asked to identify a time when their child is likely to engage in problem behaviors, and sessions are scheduled at that time. This allows live practice and feedback on the procedures. As with Tier 1 intervention, programmed home strategy sessions occur every 2 weeks to allow parents sufficient time to practice the strategies and children adequate time to respond.

Similar to Tier 1 intervention, programmed home strategies can be implemented by individuals with expertise and training in implementing behavioral interventions. Ideally, the parent education session leader continues with the families who require Tier 2 intervention. Because session leaders have already developed rapport with the family members and are familiar with their successes and difficulties with Tier 1 intervention strategies, they are able to move quickly and smoothly to Tier 2. During programmed home strategies, the leader's role becomes one of a coach to the parent(s).

The content of programmed home strategies mirrors the parent education sessions. Specifically, the following strategies are reviewed and practiced: Session 1—Attending and Rewards, Session 2—Balanced Attending and Planned Ignoring, Session 3—Point Systems and Time Out From Reinforcement, and Session 4—Planning Ahead. Session 5 is a review of the previous four coaching sessions. Parents practice techniques they had difficulty implementing correctly, and the coach and parent brainstorm ways the techniques can be generalized (e.g., implemented in community settings). The content of the remaining coaching sessions is as follows: Session 6—Transitional Warnings and When–Then Statements, Session 7—Safety in the Home, Session 8—Early Literacy, and Session 9—Early Numeracy. Session 10 consists of review and practice, similar to Session 5.

During each session, the coach begins by modeling the behavior strategy for the parent. Next, the coach lays the strategy with the parent. Parents then practice implementing the behavioral strategy with their children and receive feedback. For example, parents may be asked to describe a situation in which their child must transition from one activity to another. The parent and coach develop specific strategies for a smooth transition, such as using transitional warnings and when–then statements. The coach then demonstrates how to use the strategies, followed by parent role play. Subsequently, parents arrange situations in which their children must transition from one activity to another. The parent uses transitional warnings and when–then statements, and the coach provides feedback. Finally, parents and coach generate examples of how the strategy can be used during different situations throughout the day. This provides opportunities to address idiosyncratic home situations. For instance, if a parent has multiple children who have difficulties at bedtime, the coach and parent discuss how to stagger bedtimes, develop consistent routines, provide transitional warnings to each child, and issue when–then statements regarding the routines (e.g., "When you finish brushing your teeth, we can read books").

As with Tier 1 intervention, when Tier 2 coaching ends, responsiveness to intervention is assessed. Generally, because coaches spend a substantial amount of time in the home, they have the opportunity to observe whether Tier 2 interventions have resulted in reductions in behavior problems. For children who still do not show reductions in behavior problems following Tier 2 intervention, Tier 3 is required.


## TIER 3: ASSESSMENT-BASED INTERVENTION

Tier 3 intervention is introduced when child behavior problems continue following Tier 2 intervention. As with Tier 1, minimal or lack of improvement following Tier 2 intervention indicates the need for Tier 3 (e.g., Kern, Hilt-Panahon, & Sokol, 2009). Intervention at Tier 3 involves collecting information on the function of behavior problems (i.e., functional assessment) and then developing a related intervention plan. The functional assessment focuses on identifying *antecedents,* or events that precede problem behavior; skill deficits that may contribute to problem behavior; and consequences that may be reinforcing the problem behavior. On the basis of this information, an individualized plan can be developed that is linked to the assessment information. Tier 3 intervention is conducted in the home and should be facilitated by consultants with skill at conducting functional behavioral assessments and developing related intervention plans. Typically, weekly meetings (approximately 2 hours) are scheduled, with the process lasting 10 weeks.

During an initial meeting with parents, target behaviors that need to be decreased are collaboratively identified. When children engage in multiple problem behaviors, they should be prioritized for intervention purposes. As we described in Chapter 2, Janney and Snell (2000) provided an excellent strategy to prioritize problem behaviors. They suggested that the first priority should be *destructive* behaviors, or those that are harmful to the child or others. Examples of destructive behaviors include self-injury and aggression. The second priority for intervention is *disruptive* behavior. These behaviors do not pose an immediate danger to self or others but interfere with social, emotional, and preacademic development. In addition, behaviors that have the potential to become destructive fall into this category. Examples of disruptive behaviors are refusing to share, persistent tantrums, and declining to engage in activities. The third priority for intervention is *distracting* behaviors. Behaviors of this nature do not cause major delays in learning or social development but deviate from age-appropriate expectations for deportment. Behaviors that could become disruptive also fall within this category. Examples of distracting behaviors are excessive talking or frequently interrupting others' activities. See Table 3.1 for an overview of behavioral priorities for intervention.

After target behaviors are identified and prioritized, the consultant and parent develop operational definitions. The definitions will clarify the exact

TABLE 3.1
Hierarchy of Behaviors for Intervention

| Intervention priority | Type of behavior | Definition | Examples |
|---|---|---|---|
| High | Destructive | Behaviors harmful to self or others | Self-injury<br>Aggression |
| Moderate | Disruptive | Behaviors that interfere with development *or* may become destructive | Tantrums<br>Refusal to share<br>Failure to participate |
| Low | Distracting | Behaviors that deviate from age norms *or* may become disruptive | Excessive talking<br>Frequent interruptions |

topography of the target behavior and allow it to be measured to evaluate intervention effectiveness. For example, a parent may consider a child noncompliant if she does not follow a command immediately, whereas a consultant may believe that delay is acceptable, allowing the child time to process the instruction. Collaboratively, the parents and consultant can agree on a reasonable time delay that defines noncompliance (e.g., 5 s).

After defining the target behavior, a method should be selected to record occurrences of the behavior. Behavior can be measured using the dimensions of frequency, duration, intensity, or latency (Miltenberger, 2005). The method selected will be based on the characteristics of the target behavior. Frequency is a measure of the number of times a behavior occurs and is best matched to discrete behaviors that are brief in length. Hitting a sibling or grabbing his or her toy are examples of behaviors that are well suited to frequency measurement. Behaviors that tend to endure over a period of time are best measured using duration. Specifically, the duration of time that a behavior occurs is measured from start to end. Behaviors such as tantrums or out of seat are generally measured using duration. The intensity of a behavior can also be measured, particularly if the goal is not to eliminate the behavior but to change its form. An example of a target behavior suitable for an intensity measure is a child's inappropriate voice volume, such as yelling or screaming. The goal is not to eliminate talk but to reduce the volume. Categories of vocalization intensity can be established, such as 3 = *yelling or screaming at an extremely loud volume*, 2 = *talking at a volume that is slightly louder than conversational level*, and 1 = *talking at a volume that is conversational level*. Finally, latency measures how long it takes a child to initiate behavior following a prompt. This is an appropriate measure for behaviors such as difficulty following directions or complying after the first instruction, which are characteristic of young children with ADHD. The time between when an instruction is issued (e.g., "Come to the dinner table") and when the child initiates the behavior in accordance with the instruction (e.g., begins walking toward the table) is measured.

Because most parents are unfamiliar and inexperienced with data collection, it is generally best to design simple strategies. For example, if parents are measuring the frequency of a behavior, they can be given a golf counter to attach to a belt loop. Each time the behavior occurs, they simply press a button on the counter. At the end of a designated period of time (e.g., after school hours), they can record the number on the golf counter corresponding to the behavior's frequency. For duration measures, rather than recording the exact time a behavior starts and ends, a data collection sheet can be developed that is divided into intervals (e.g., 10 minutes, 15 minutes). Parents can then indicate with a checkmark whether the behavior occurred during that interval. Although this procedure does not provide an exact measure of behavior duration, it offers an approximation. Similarly, parents can estimate the latency to behavior by silently counting (e.g., "one one-thousand, two one-thousand") and record a latency approximation.

When there is consensus on the problem behavior that will be targeted for intervention and its measurement, functional assessment information is gathered. Information gathering takes two formats: indirect and direct. Indirect methods are used at times other than when problem behavior is occurring and rely on parent recall, whereas direct methods of information gathering are used when the behavior in actually occurring, through direct observation.

The purpose of both indirect and direct methods is to obtain information that will directly contribute to intervention development. In addition to data on the occurrence of behavior problems, four other types of information are pertinent for a functional assessment-based intervention (Kern, O'Neill, & Starosta, 2005). The first is antecedents, which are events that precede the problem behavior. Antecedents have been referred to as *fast triggers* in that they occur just before and elicit problem behavior. Antecedents may include a request to perform a task (e.g., "Brush your teeth," "Clean up your toys"), restricted access to something desirable (e.g., removal of a toy, termination of a preferred activity), or the absence of attention (e.g., parent is helping a sibling with homework).

The second type of information gathered is consequences, or events that follow problem behavior. Often, parents respond to behavior in some way that inadvertently provides reinforcement for the behavior. For example, it is not uncommon for parents to withdraw a demand when their child engages in problem behavior. This type of information is important to determine what type of parent behavior (i.e., reinforcement) may function to maintain child behavior.

Consequences are generally considered with respect to the way they function to reinforce problem behavior, rather than the specific topography of the response (Iwata, Dorsey, Slifer, Bauman, & Richman, 1982). The reinforcing function of problem behavior generally falls into two broad categories consistent with positive and negative reinforcement paradigms (Skinner, 1953). In the first category is *positive reinforcement,* which is behavior that occurs to obtain something desirable, such as attention or a tangible item or activity. For instance, when a parent is interacting with a sibling, the child with ADHD may tantrum to interrupt the interaction and obtain her parent's attention. Unable to continue the sibling interaction, the parent may attempt to stop the child from engaging in the tantrum, thereby reinforcing the problem behavior by providing attention. In the case of a tangible function, a child may impulsively grab toys away from his sibling. To avoid further problems, the sibling may allow her brother to have the toy. In this manner, grabbing the toy has been reinforced through access to the item.

The second broad category is *negative reinforcement,* which is behavior that occurs to escape something undesirable. For young children with ADHD, escape typically occurs in the context of a difficult or nonpreferred task. In home settings, tasks that are typically problematic for children with ADHD include sitting and behaving at the dinner table, completing bedtime routines and going to bed, and performing lengthy or multistep tasks (e.g., cleaning a room of toys). When a parent's request to complete a task is followed by problem behavior and the parent does not persist with the task requirement, the problem behavior is reinforced through escape from the task.

In addition to information about antecedents and consequences, a third type of information parents are asked about is skill deficits that may contribute to the problem behavior (e.g., Halle, Bambara, & Reichle, 2005). Skill deficits may involve fine or gross motor skills necessary to complete a task, difficulties with language, lack of sustained attention needed to complete an activity, or problems with social skills necessary to get along with siblings and peers. To reduce problem behavior over the long term, it is important to ensure that children are taught new skills that they can use in situations that are problematic. For example, children must learn how to ask their parents for help when they are unable to complete a task independently. Likewise, children must be able to ask their sibling for a turn, rather than grabbing a toy.

Finally, the fourth type of information parents are asked about is distal events (also referred to as *setting events* or *establishing operations*) that may indirectly contribute to problem behavior (Michael, 1993). *Distal events* are those that do not directly cause problem behavior but increase the probability that problem behavior will occur in the presence of particular antecedents. For example, asking a child to set the table (antecedent) when the child is tired (setting event) may lead to a tantrum. Generally, the request to set the table is met with child compliance except in the particular setting event of fatigue. When the antecedents to problem behavior are intermittently associated with problem behavior, setting events or establishing operations should be considered (e.g., Kennedy & Meyer, 1996). See Table 3.2 for a description and examples of information relevant for a functional assessment.

At the initial parent meeting, the home-based functional assessment process is initiated, beginning with a parent interview. During this interview, parents are asked to identify potential antecedents to and consequences of problem behavior as well as distal events that may play a role in child problem behavior. In addition, any child skill deficits are identified. A number of structured interviews are available to guide the interview process (e.g., Bambara & Kern, 2005; Kratochwill & Bergan, 1990; O'Neill, Horner, Albin, Sprague, Storey, & Newton, 1997).

During the second parent meeting, parents are taught to use an antecedent–behavior–consequence (ABC) format to collect information

TABLE 3.2
Information Relevant for a Functional Assessment

| Type of information | Definition | Examples |
|---|---|---|
| Antecedents | Events that precede problem behavior | Instruction to put toys away<br>Requirement to sit at dinner time<br>Parent busy with sibling, so attention unavailable<br>Toy taken away by sibling |
| Consequences | Events that follow problem behavior | Demand removed following tantrum<br>Attention given following disruption<br>Toy provided following aggression |
| Skill deficits | Lack of skills that may contribute to problem behavior | Difficulty attending for longer than 3 minutes<br>Inability to request play item appropriately<br>Problems waiting for turn |
| Distal events | Events that occur at an earlier time and increase the likelihood of problem behavior in the presence of particular antecedents | Lack of sleep<br>Hunger<br>Illness |

about events associated with problem behavior. In other words, parents are asked to collect data on events that occur before problem behavior (A or antecedents), behavior (B), and the events that follow problem behavior (C or consequences). The consultant describes situations in which problem behavior may occur while the parent practices collecting data using the ABC format. In our experience, most parents have little difficulty collecting ABC data. Parents are asked to complete ABC direct observation data collection daily for at least a week.

During the subsequent visit, the consultant conducts a 2-hour naturalistic direct observation in the home, noting problem behavior, antecedents, and consequences. These data are used to supplement parent-collected data.

During Session 4, the parent conducts an analogue brief functional analysis (e.g., Northup et al., 1991), with prompting and coaching from the consultant throughout. Specifically, four 5-minute sessions are arranged and presented in random order, with at least 10 minutes between sessions. Sessions consist of *control* (play), in which the parent engages in preferred activities with the child and refrains from issuing demands; *task*, in which the child is asked to complete a task (e.g., put toys away, brush teeth); *attention*, in which the child is asked to play independently while parent attention is diverted; and *tangible*, in which access to a preferred toy or activity is restricted. Contingent on problem behavior, reinforcement respective to the assessment condition is provided (i.e., escape, attention, or access). For example, in the tangible condition, if the child engages in problem behavior, then access to the preferred toy or activity is briefly restricted. After the four sessions are completed, all sessions with high rates of problem behavior are replicated, alternating with sessions with low rates of problem behavior. The results of this analogue functional analysis suggest situations that may be associated with problem behavior in naturalistic settings and consequences that may reinforce the problem behavior. The replication is designed to provide further evidence of variables (antecedents and consequences) associated with problem behavior.

A functional analysis was conducted with Kyle, a 4-year-old boy considered to be at risk for ADHD. Kyle's parents were concerned because he engaged in aggression toward both of them at home. They attended parent education and received Tier 2 home coaching. Kyle's parents faithfully implemented the interventions they learned during parent education and coaching at home. Although the interventions reduced Kyle's aggression from approximately 20 per day to about 10 per day, the rate of his continued aggression was unacceptable. Thus, it was decided that a Tier 3 assessment-based intervention was needed to further identify the function of Kyle's aggression and develop a more specific and individualized intervention plan.

The results of Kyle's home-based functional analysis are shown in Figure 3.2. The initial session was escape, during which he exhibited high-rate aggressions at 36 per hour (three aggressions during the 5-minute session). Aggression was very low or absent during the subsequent three sessions (play, tangible, attention). To confirm the function, the escape session was repli-

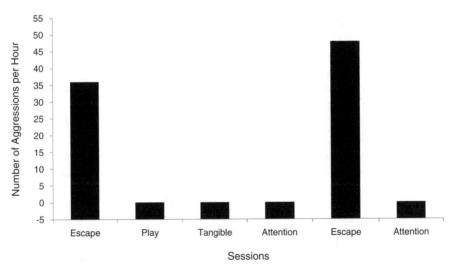

*Figure 3.2.* Home-based functional analysis for Kyle.

cated, alternating with attention. During the replication, escape again resulted in a rate of 48 aggressions per hour, and no problem behavior was observed during the attention session. Thus, the functional analysis indicated that escape was the function of Kyle's aggression.

After the interview, parent-collected ABC data, consultant observation, and analogue functional analysis are completed, and the data are summarized to determine the variables (antecedents, consequences) related to problem behavior as well as skill deficits and setting events that might influence the occurrence of problem behavior. The consultant reviews each data source to evaluate convergence, consistency, or the need for alternate interventions on the basis of unique findings from the assessments (i.e., parent-collected data indicating problem behaviors at the grocery).

It should be noted that problem behavior frequently occurs for more than one reason. In other words, problem behavior may serve multiple functions. In an examination of home-based functional analysis data from 42 preschool children who participated in our larger study (Kern et al., 2007), multiple functions were identified for 55%, or 23 children (Sokol, Kern, Arbolino, Thomas, & DuPaul, 2009). Overall, escape was the primary function for 35 children. This was followed by a tangible function for 24 children. An attention function occurred least frequently, observed in 13 children. When problem behavior had multiple functions, escape was almost always one of the functions (occurring for 22 of the 23 participants), whereas tangible was one of the functions for 19 of the 23 participants.

During Session 5, the consultant meets with the parent, and they jointly review the assessment findings, conferring until agreement is reached on the antecedents, consequences and function of problem behavior, skill deficits, and setting events. Hypothesis statements that summarize the assessment data and serve as a link between assessment information and intervention are jointly developed. Hypothesis statements identify the antecedent, problem behavior, and presumed function and, when relevant, also describe a setting event. An example of a hypothesis statement is, "When Derek is asked to clean his room (antecedent), he tantrums (problem behavior) to escape the task (function)." Another example is, "When Jennifer's mother sits down to help Jennifer's sister with homework (antecedent), Jennifer engages in aggression (problem behavior) to get her mother's attention (function)." A hypothesis statement that includes a setting event is, "When Hakim did not sleep well (setting event) and he is told to dress for school (antecedent), he yells and screams (problem behavior) to escape the task (function)." In addition to developing hypothesis statements, the consultant discusses potential interventions with the parents.

During the week that follows, the consultant develops an intervention plan for the family. The plan consists of antecedent strategies to prevent problem behavior, instructional techniques to address skill deficits (e.g., social interaction problems, waiting) and replacement behaviors (e.g., appropriately requesting a break or soliciting attention), consequences for problem behavior that are unlikely to reinforce the behavior, and ways to eliminate or ameliorate setting events (for additional detail about intervention components, see Chapter 4). During Session 6, the consultant provides the parent with a fully developed, assessment-based, individualized, multicomponent intervention plan. The parents and consultant review the plan and make additions or modifications as needed to address parent preference, potential effectiveness, and implementation feasibility. The consultant models each intervention strategy, role-plays with the parent, and observes parents implementing the strategy with their children while providing feedback.

Remaining home visits focus on further coaching and feedback on implementation of the individualized intervention plan. Additional modeling and role play takes place as needed, indicated by parent report of challenges and observed parent skill implementing the interventions. Generally, four additional sessions are sufficient for most parents to implement the plan with integrity and consistency.

## EVALUATING PROGRESS

Parent-collected data on the target behavior gathered before implementing the intervention (e.g., during ABC data collection) serves as a baseline comparison with data collected after the intervention is implemented. When evaluating child progress, it is important to keep in mind that it takes time for parents to change the way they interact with their children, and it takes time for children to learn new and appropriate ways of behaving. Hence, behavior may change slowly. It is most imperative that behavior problems are continuing to decline. Parents often do not notice change in behavior when it is gradual. Thus, it is helpful to provide parents with graphic displays depicting behavior change. Seeing data in graphic form encourages parents that behavior is likely to continue to improve.

When improvements occur, the plan should be maintained until behavior change is durable. That is, reductions in problem behavior should be maintained over a sufficient period of time to indicate that children have learned alternative strategies to get their needs met and problem behavior is no longer necessary. This generally takes several months, but it may take more or less time depending on the severity of the behavior problem and the consistency of intervention implementation. After behavioral improvements have been maintained over a sufficient period of time, intervention fading should be considered. Fading is important for several reasons. First, interventions are sometimes stigmatizing in that supports are in place that are not typically implemented with the child's same-age peers. For instance, self-monitoring appropriate peer play at 5-minute intervals causes interruptions from the ongoing activity and may draw unwanted attention to the child. Another reason fading is important is that intervention can be labor-intensive to implement. Parents are often relieved to know that long-term plans are in place to decrease the intensity of the intervention.

Intervention fading is most successful when it is done gradually and systematically (e.g., Rock & Thead, 2007). When fading is gradual and systematic, children do not notice changes, and behavior reductions are more likely to be sustained. For example, Savannah had extreme difficulties sustaining her attention when her mother read books to her. At the initiation of intervention, she was able to sit in her seat and attend for no more than a few minutes before becoming fidgety and distracted. Thus, in addition to letting her choose a book for nightly reading, her mother initially read one very short book that could be completed in no more than 3 minutes. Within a month, Savannah was attending well during the brief reading session, so her mother began fading intervention by gradually increasing the length of reading time. She purchased longer books and read for 4 minutes each night. As long as Savannah was able to attend throughout the reading session at least 6 of 7 nights during the week, her mother increased reading time by 1 minute. Within 4 months, Savannah was able to attend to stories for 15 minutes. This helped her at school as well, where a daily 10- to 15-minute story time was scheduled.

If problem behavior does not decline, the first step should be to assess whether parents are implementing the plan as it was designed and on a consistent basis. If treatment adherence is not occurring at a sufficient level, it is important to assess why parents are not implementing the plan. It may be that they do not fully understand how to implement the strategies and need additional coaching. Alternatively, the plan may not be feasible for the parent to implement for reasons such as competing responsibilities in the home. In this case, the plan needs to be revised to better accommodate the home context. If the plan is being implemented consistently as designed, it may be that the hypotheses regarding problem behavior were not accurate. In these situations, it may be necessary to collect additional functional behavioral assessment data to develop new hypotheses and revise the support plan.

## HOME-BASED INTERVENTION CASE EXAMPLE

Adrian was a 4-year-old boy diagnosed with ADHD—combined type. His mother indicated that from birth he was far more active than her other two children. Difficulties with both inattention and impulsivity–hyperactivity were confirmed during an initial psychological evaluation. Mr. and Mrs. R. faithfully attended Tier 1 parent education sessions but reported little change in Adrian's behavior. Subsequently, Tier 2 home-based coaching was completed, still with insufficient behavioral improvements. Thus, Tier 3, assessment-based intervention was initiated with Adrian.

Tier 3 intervention began with a meeting with Mr. and Mrs. R., with the goal of identifying Adrian's problem behavior and conducting an initial interview. Adrian's parents were clear that noncompliance and tantrums were Adrian's major problems. During the initial interview, they indicated that they had difficulty getting Adrian to follow almost any instruction. They admitted that although they understood how to follow through, sometimes it was too difficult because of Adrian's tantrums and the time it takes away from their other children. They also stated that he has difficulties with his siblings, usually because he refused to share his toys or took his siblings toys from their rooms. In response to these sibling problems, his parents sent him to his room for time out.

During the following week, Adrian's parents recorded the frequency of Adrian's noncompliance and both the frequency and duration of his tantrums. The data indicated that problem behaviors occurred several times daily, with noncompliance occurring three to eight times a day and tantrums occurring two to four times each day. Subsequently, Mr. and Mrs. R. collected ABC data, noting the events that occurred just before noncompliance and tantrums and the events that followed. The ABC data were indeed consistent with the interview information, indicating that problem behavior occurred regularly when given particular instructions. Specifically, noncompliance and tantrums were noted every night when Adrian was told it was bedtime. In addition, noncompliance also occurred during cleanup tasks, usually when he was asked to put away his toys. In addition, as the parents reported in the interview, one or more tantrums occurred daily when Mrs. R. was preparing dinner and the children were playing.

The consultant then conducted a home-based observation, collecting data on occurrences of noncompliance and tantrums as well as the events that preceded and followed problem behavior. Adrian's problem behavior was less frequent in her presence; however, her observation concurred with the parent reports and ABC data regarding antecedents and consequences. That is, problem behavior occurred around demands (particularly bedtime) and during play, when he refused to share and grabbed toys from his siblings. She also noted that bedtime was particularly chaotic, and it took more than 45 minutes to get Adrian to bed. In addition, although Adrian was once sent to time out for "not playing nicely," more often his siblings acquiesced to his behavior, allowing him to play alone or giving up their toys on his demand.

Following the naturalistic observation, an analog functional analysis was conducted. The findings, shown in Figure 3.3, indicated that the function for Adrian's behavior was both escape and tangible. Together, the findings from all of the assessments pointed to escape and tangible functions. Further, it appeared that Adrian's related behavior resulted from unclear or ambiguous expectations, whereas his tangible problem behavior was related to difficulties sharing. Thus, two hypotheses were developed. The first stated, "When instructions are inconsistent or ambiguous, Adrian engages in problem behavior to escape the demand." The second hypothesis stated, "When Adrian is required to share toys, he engages in problem behavior to obtain or maintain access to the toy."

With information about the specific circumstances associated with Adrian's problem behavior, an individualized support plan was developed. Table 3.3 shows the supports that were introduced to reduce Adrian's problem behavior, including antecedent modifications, skill instruction, and consequences. Distinct interventions were developed to address problem behavior related to each function (escape, tangible). The plan resulted in immediate reductions in tantrums and noncompliance, which continued further as Adrian became more fluent with the alternative skills he was taught.

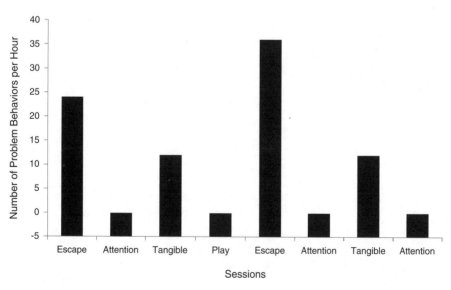

*Figure 3.3.* Home-based functional analysis for Adrian.

## TABLE 3.3
### Adrian's Behavior Support Plan

| Antecedent interventions | Skill instruction | Consequences |
|---|---|---|
| Hypothesis 1: When instructions are inconsistent or ambiguous, Adrian engages in problem behavior to escape the demand. | | |
| Stagger bedtimes for each child | Teach Adrian to ask, "What should I do next?" when he is unclear about routine | Ignore inappropriate behavior and follow through with routine |
| Establish consistent bedtime for Adrian (8 p.m.) | | |
| Develop consistent nighttime routine (brush teeth, wash face, go to bathroom); develop picture schedule, and provide reward for following routine | Teach Adrian to follow schedule independently | Provide reminders of reward for following routine and extra reading time |
| End routine with enjoyable activity (reading in bed) and allow an extra 5 minutes of reading if Adrian completes routine and is in bed within 10 minutes | | |
| Hypothesis 2: When Adrian is required to share toys, he engages in problem behavior to obtain or maintain access to the toy. | | |
| Prepractice sharing with siblings (each day before play, model and practice turn taking) | | |
| Supervise sibling playtime for at least 15 minutes daily; schedule an activity that requires turn taking, and praise children for appropriately taking turns | | |

## CONCLUSIONS

Home-based intervention is critical given the important and substantial role parents play in their young child's development and behavior. A tiered approach to home-based intervention has been demonstrated to be effective and cost- and labor-efficient. At Tier 1, behavioral concepts and procedures can be taught in a group context. Tier 2 offers an increased level of support in the home, through practice and coaching. Many young children with ADHD symptoms respond to Tiers 1 and 2 intervention and do not require the intensive, individualized support that occurs at Tier 3. Support at Tier 3 involves a home-based plan derived from functional assessment and functional analysis information. Such a plan is developed in collaboration with parents and involves interventions that prevent problem behavior, provide skill instruction, and implement strategies to respond to problem behavior.

There are challenges that may be encountered when implementing the approach described in this chapter. Common challenges and potential solutions are described in Exhibit 3.1.

EXHIBIT 3.1
Challenges to Implementation

---

*Issue: Our preschool is offering parent education classes. Several parents are complaining that it is too difficult to remember to implement rewards for appropriate behavior and praise. They report that they frequently fall back into old habits, such as yelling at their child.*

Potential solution: Just as it is sometimes difficult to change child behavior, adults also have difficulty changing their behavior. This is particularly true when emotions are involved, such as when they are feeling angry or frustrated with their child's behavior. Often it is helpful to have parents self-monitor their behavior. For example, a parent can keep track of the number of times she praises her child throughout the day and aim for slightly higher rates each day. Similarly, parents can self-monitor their responses to their child's problem behavior, such as noting when they ignored or redirected the behavior rather than yelling at the child. Also, it is important to continue to remind parents that the techniques they used in the past did not lead to reductions in problem behavior, emphasizing the importance of modifying their behavior to change their child's behavior.

*Issue: I am working with a parent to implement an assessment-based plan. I have noticed reductions in her child's problem behavior, but the parent insists that the child has not changed.*

Potential solution: Sometimes behavior problem reduction is slow, particularly if a child needs to learn new skills that are not already a part of his or her repertoire, such as asking for help. In these situations, it is important to collect data so that the parent can see that behavior problems are decreasing. Parents can collect data themselves, or therapists can collect data during home visits. Graphic displays of data can help parents visually see their child's behavior improvements.

*Issue: As a clinician, I am unable to make frequent home visits to implement Tier 2 or 3 interventions. Are there any alternatives?*

Potential alternatives: Home visits are optimal because they allow clinicians to observe the child and family under naturally occurring situations. However, when this is not possible, coaching can occur in a clinic setting. Situations can be arranged to replicate what typically happens at home (e.g., the child is required to pick up toys), and parents practice strategies to address problem behaviors during those situations. Another alternative is for parents to videotape problematic situations in the home. The clinician may be able identify behavioral function using the videotapes and can provide the parent with feedback about his or her interactions with the child and responses to the child's problem behaviors. In addition, analog functional analysis can be conducted in a clinic setting. Although it is difficult to replicate the variables and conditions that occur at home, a function can often be identified that assists with intervention development.

---

# 4

# PRESCHOOL-BASED BEHAVIORAL
# INTERVENTION STRATEGIES

For most young children, preschool or day care is the first structured setting where they spend substantial amounts time learning and interacting with their peers. The preschool years are a critical time when children begin to develop the social and preacademic skills that serve as the foundation for future development. Research has shown that young children with established social and academic readiness skills fare much better throughout their academic career than do children with early deficits in these areas (Campbell & Ewing, 1990; Dishion, French, & Patterson, 1996; Hinshaw & Anderson, 1996). Hence, the preschool years represent an opportune time to ensure that children are fully prepared for the years ahead.

Research indicates that an increasing number of children enter preschool with social, emotional, and behavioral problems. Estimates of the specific number vary from study to study. For instance, Campbell (1995) estimated that 10% to 15% of preschool age children exhibit mild to moderate behavior problems, similar to the rates identified by the Early Childhood Longitudinal Study (West, Denton, & Germino-Hausken, 2000). More concerning, Lavigne et al. (1996) found that 21% of preschoolers met diagnostic criteria for a disorder because of their behavior problems, and the symptoms of 9% of children could be classified as severe. These data indicate that preschool teachers and day care providers must not only be prepared to organize the routine experiences that set the stage for later learning but also be skilled at addressing the complex social, behavioral, and learning problems present in the current population of young children.

Unfortunately, many preschool and day care teachers indicate that they do not feel equipped to handle the social and behavioral problems of the children in their classrooms (Walter, Gouze, & Lim, 2006). Teachers report that they spend a great deal of time addressing behavior problems, which consequently impinges on instructional time. Research underscores the significant problem this poses in early education settings. For example, in a survey of more than 500 early-childhood educators, the training need rated highest was addressing problem behavior (Hemeter, Corso, & Cheatham, 2006). One direct consequence of inadequate skills to reduce problem behavior was identified in a study by W. S. Gilliam (2005), which found that young children are expelled from preschool programs at 3 times the rate of students in kindergarten through Grade 12. It is likely that many, if not most, of these children exhibit early symptoms of attention-deficit/hyperactivity disorder (ADHD). Regrettably, expulsion from preschool means they do not have the opportunity to learn the important social and behavioral repertoires that will be required for the remainder of their educational years, nor will they be exposed to important preacademic skills.

Fortunately, as we mentioned in Chapter 2, new models of support are relatively easy to implement and make behavior management and preacademic instruction feasible in preschool settings. Further, the tiered organization of these models ensures that all children will receive support, with intensity matched to need. In this chapter, we describe a tiered model of support for preschool and day care settings. Although the interventions are applicable for all students, we focus primarily on behavior problems that young children with or at risk for ADHD are likely to exhibit, particularly at Tier 3.

## OVERVIEW OF PRESCHOOL MODEL

There are several benefits to establishing a model of behavior management or support in preschool or day care environments. First, increasing numbers of children are entering early-education settings with social and emotional difficulties that require intervention. Second, identification of early symptoms of disabilities and disorders is improving, suggesting children who will benefit from proactive strategies to prevent the worsening of symptoms. Finally, social, emotional, behavioral, and learning problems are best remediated with early intervention. For these reasons, it is increasingly important that children receive the supports they need as soon as they enter preschool or day care.

Given the increased needs among the general population of young children, strategies that teach and promote appropriate behavior to *all* children are considered most beneficial (Fox, Dunlap, Hemmeter, Joseph, & Strain, 2003). In most preschool settings, this level of universal support is likely to address the needs of the majority of children. For those who are nonresponsive to this type of universal intervention, additional supports can be provided.

As we have noted in earlier chapters, a model of tiered support has many benefits. One is that it is both cost- and time-efficient. Specifically, when behavior is managed effectively on a classwide basis, resources are available for the few students who require increasingly intensive supports. Thus, rather than attempting to address the behavior problems of numerous children in a classroom, fewer resources will be needed for the few nonresponsive students who need individualized programs. In addition, the model focuses on prevention. That is, instruction is provided followed by modeling and practicing new skills. Most behavior problems can be prevented through this type of systematic teaching. Finally, staff members are consistent in the way they respond to children, with respect to both reinforcing appropriate behavior and responding to inappropriate behavior.

The model of support we describe herein involves three tiers (see Figure 4.1). Tier 1, or *universal intervention*, is used on a classwide basis—that is, all children receive intervention. In preschool programs with multiple classrooms, such as Head Start, Tier 1 intervention can be implemented buildingwide. Implementing Tier 1 intervention has the benefit of establishing consistent child expectations. This consistency is advantageous when children are gathered in cross-class groups, when they are in common areas (e.g., hallways), or when they switch classrooms within the academic year or from year to year. In addition, staff members benefit by understanding the expectations for all children. In this way, monitoring is improved, and consequences are consistently applied. Finally, with a single, buildingwide approach, staff training is facilitated. All staff members can be trained simultaneously, colleagues can work together and support one another with implementation, and supervisors understand the consistent procedures across all classrooms in the building.

Tier 2, or *small-group skill instruction*, is introduced for children who do not respond to Tier 1 interventions. Support at this level is generally provided for small groups of children. Because it is implemented in small groups, it is not extraordinarily costly or time-consuming. When the model is implemented buildingwide, children from multiple classrooms can be grouped for instruction, further reducing the overall time and cost.

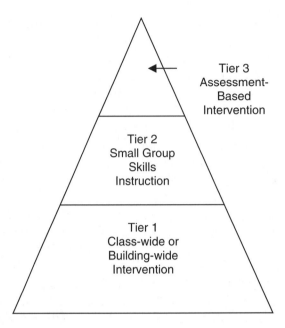

*Figure 4.1.* Illustration of tiered support at preschool for young children with attention-deficit/hyperactivity disorder.

When Tiers 1 and 2 are implemented successfully, few children should require Tier 3, or *assessment-based intervention*. Tier 3 intervention requires collecting assessment information and developing and implementing an individualized plan, making it fairly labor-intensive. In most early intervention settings, only one or two children will require Tier 3 intervention, provided Tiers 1 and 2 interventions are well designed and implemented.

GETTING STARTED

Establishing a system of positive and proactive supports requires preparation and planning. Teachers often are accustomed to addressing problem behavior after it occurs, rather than designing systems of prevention. In addition, adults tend to use punitive procedures with children and rarely employ a range of options. Further, sometimes teachers have the expectation that children should enter preschool already knowing how to behave and are not inclined to take the time to teach appropriate behavior. Thus, it is essential for teachers to understand the benefits of a tiered approach and what is expected of them. When buy-in is obtained in advance, implementation is facilitated.

Obtaining buy-in requires that teachers understand the philosophy of a tiered approach that focuses on instruction and prevention and agree to its implementation. In buildings implementing tiered support, leadership teams are generally established to develop an implementation plan, determine training needs, monitor progress, and address ongoing needs and issues that arise. The team generally includes someone with expertise in behavior problems (e.g., behavior specialist, mental health worker, disability coordinator), along with a teacher, parent, and administrator. Teams meet regularly (e.g., monthly) to plan and coordinate. When a single classroom is implementing a tiered model, the team may consist of the full classroom teaching staff. If no one has expertise in behavioral issues, consultation is recommended.

When initiating a tiered model of prevention, the first step is to obtain commitment from staff members. It is suggested that at least 80% of staff members agree to change their behavior management approach and implement preventive interventions (Horner & Sugai, 2000). Team members, the classroom individual initiating the change, or a consultant provide staff members with information regarding the rationale and benefits of such an approach. There are many websites and materials available to facilitate this process (e.g., http://www.PBIS.org; http://www.osepideasthatwork.org/toolkit/pdf/SchoolwideBehaviorSupport.pdf). After staff members fully understand the model and what will be expected and the majority of them agree to implementation, training in each tier can be initiated.

## TIER 1 UNIVERSAL INTERVENTION

Tier 1 intervention for preschool or day care settings involves establishing and teaching expectations, with a particular focus on behavioral deportment and interpersonal relations, (e.g., Fox, Jack, & Broyles, 2005). All children in a preschool or day care classroom or program receive Tier 1 intervention. This level is designed to teach and encourage behavior appropriate to the setting, including prosocial peer and adult interactions, and to enhance children's understanding and appropriate expression of their emotions.

At this tier, classwide or programwide expectations are developed, accompanied by reinforcement for adhering to expectations and consistent consequences for failing to adhere to expectations. Rules that are developmentally appropriate for preschool-age children must be simple and few in number (e.g., three to five). Further, rules are stated positively so that they teach children what behavior is expected. Examples of a program's rules are *Be Nice to Others*, *Take Turns*, and *Keep Hands and Feet to Yourself*. To implement rules consistently, all staff must agree on operational definitions. For instance, *Be Nice to Others* may include "using only kind words with classmates and staff, listening when others are talking, and helping each other with activities and tasks." The expectations should be posted in a prominent location, accompanied by drawings to facilitate understanding for nonreaders.

A system of reinforcement and consequences is also developed, both to encourage appropriate behavior and to ensure that all staff members respond to infractions consistently. Because the focus is on teaching children how to behave appropriately, the reinforcement provided for adhering to expectations must be most salient. General guidelines suggest a ratio of at least three to four statements acknowledging appropriate behavior for every one corrective statement. Young children respond well to praise, so verbal public recognition is usually sufficient. In more difficult classrooms, a token economy, such as a star chart, can be developed in which children receive the choice of a small, tangible item or privilege (e.g., sitting with the teacher at lunch) for earning a predetermined number of tokens or stars. In addition, tokens can be placed in a jar, and then weekly or monthly drawings may be held for a larger prize. This type of reward recognizes children in a public way, further promoting and acknowledging appropriate behavior.

In addition to providing rewards for following the expectations, consequences for not following the expectations should be established. Consequences that are natural or logical help children understand the connection between their behavior and its results. In addition, consequences can be arranged so that they are instructive. For example, if Gina calls Rafael a derogatory name, she may be asked to apologize to him to facilitate her understanding of his hurt feelings and to pay him a compliment, which teaches her an appropriate interaction. Consequences also should be age-appropriate. For example, a brief time out may effectively reduce behavior that is attention seeking, but it should be no longer than a couple of minutes.

After rules have been developed along with their associated rewards and consequences, all staff members in a classroom or building must fully understand the system. Early research demonstrated that inconsistent reinforcement or consequences can make inappropriate behavior extremely durable (Ferster & Skinner, 1957). Thus, consistency is an important part of the system and encourages a rapid understanding of what is expected in the preschool setting. In larger buildings, staff members outside of the classroom have occasional opportunities to interact with children in the office, on the playground, or other common locations. It is important for those staff members (e.g., secretaries, playground monitors) to understand the expectations fully and how they are to respond to appropriate and inappropriate behaviors. Generally, the full staff is gathered before the start of an "academic year" for training purposes. The expectations and consequences are reviewed and clarified.

Subsequently, the system is introduced to children. In addition to being taught the expectations, children need to be taught the behaviors consistent with those expectations. This differs from prior approaches in which it was assumed that children came to preschool knowing behavioral expectations. Instead, it is assumed that children may not know how to behave in a preschool setting and require explicit instruction. To teach children the behavior associated with each expectation, examples and nonexamples are provided. For example, staff members may describe what it means to take turns with equipment and toys during playtime on the playground and with activities and at centers in the classroom. Staff members engage in role play with children, then children practice with one another to enhance understanding. For example, a staff member may demonstrate how to share a toy with a child, then pairs of children may be given a toy to practice turn taking.

Subsequently, following rules is practiced in vivo. Practice in the actual setting greatly increases display of the expected behavior (Lewis, Sugai, & Colvin, 1998). Practice is particularly important for young children with or at risk for ADHD who may understand the rules or expectations but have difficulties with adherence because of impulsivity. In vivo instruction begins with prepractice. This involves identifying potentially problematic situations, reciting the applicable rule, and practicing the associated behavior just before the activity. For example, if a few children are observed to have difficulty waiting for their turn on a new playground slide, a staff member may state, "Remember the rule *Take Turns* when you are on the playground. This means you go to the back of the line after you take your turn. Then you wait until all of the children in line have had their turn before you take another. Now, show me what it means to go to the back of the line and wait your turn." Then, when outside playtime begins, children are periodically reminded to take turns and praised when they are observed doing so.

Children also need to be familiar with the reward and consequence system. Most important, staff members must stress that they will be looking for appropriate behavior and rewarding children accordingly. This will reinforce the notion that the system is designed to teach and encourage children to interact appropriately and to get along with others. In addition, they should be taught the consequences for failing to adhere to the expectations. This will help them view the system as fair and consistent.

## TIER 2: SMALL-GROUP SKILLS INSTRUCTION

Tier 2 intervention is designed for children who continue to engage in problem behavior after Tier 1 intervention has been in place. Tier 2 support generally consists of small-group instruction that is linked to a specific skill. Children are grouped for instruction according to the nature of the problem behaviors they continue to exhibit. Small groups may comprise a few students in the classroom or, in the case of center-based intervention, students across classrooms. Also, support at this level can take the form of a program to increase attention to children or enhance home–school communication.

An example of a Tier 2 intervention is small-group instruction on interaction skills. It is common for a few children in a classroom to have ongoing difficulties with peer interactions for a number of reasons, such as a lack of prior experience interacting with same-age peers or the acceptance of aggressive behavior with siblings at home. Small groups may be gathered two or three times a week for additional practice. Role play should focus on particular difficulties the children have experienced. For example, if a child has difficulty getting along with others because he must be "in charge" and will not allow others a turn at being the leader, instruction may consist of reviewing why people enjoy being the leader of a game and discussing the roles of those who are not leaders. For example, when playing "follow the leader," children may describe why they enjoy being the leader and how they behave when they are not leader (e.g., wait for the leader and the persons in front of you to move, copy what they have done). Children also can be taught a strategy for coping with their anger or disappointment when they cannot be leader. This may take the form of self-instruction, such as stating to oneself, "It is OK, I will be leader soon." Children then practice taking turns being the leader and the follower in their small groups.

Another type of Tier 2 intervention involves "Check in Check Out" (Hawken, MacLeod, & Rawlings, 2007). This program involves identifying an adult, such as a classroom aide, to check in with the child each morning, periodically throughout the day, and each afternoon before going home. Typically, a point card is developed for the child with expectations associated with particular areas of difficulty. For instance, an expectation for a child who frequently calls others disparaging names might state, "I will say only kind words to others." The classroom teacher then monitors the child's peer interactions during brief intervals of time (e.g., every 15 minute), providing points for intervals with appropriate interactions. Periodically, the adult assigned to oversee the program checks in with the child, providing praise for intervals with appropriate interactions and encouragement to continue to interact appropriately with peers. This intervention may be particularly effective for children who enjoy adult attention.

Daily report cards are another type of Tier 2 intervention. These involve designing a home–school communication strategy. The purpose of this type of program is for children to receive additional rewards at home for appropriate school behavior. It is not designed as a punitive procedure in which children are punished at home for school transgressions. The simplest format is a checklist that teachers complete at the end of the day. The checklist contains targeted skills for the child, such as "Amanda followed the classroom rules."

An associated evaluative point system is designed. For example, a happy face may mean that Amanda followed all of the rules, a neutral face translates to following the rules all but one or two times, and a sad face indicates that Amanda had three or more rule infractions. Arrangements for reinforcement at home can be made when the system is developed. The reinforcement schedule should begin in such a way that it is easy to achieve at the start. For example, if Amanda has great difficulties following the rules, she may be expected to receive neutral faces at least 4 of 5 school days to earn a special privilege on the weekend. This can be modified to include at least one happy face as Amanda's behavior improves.

## TIER 3: ASSESSMENT-BASED INTERVENTION

Tier 3 intervention is needed for children who do not respond to Tiers 1 and 2 intervention. Also, for children who engage in severe problem behavior, Tier 3 intervention can be introduced immediately (see Chapter 2 for a discussion of the circumstances that dictate such action). In most classrooms, only one or two children will require Tier 3 intervention. Consistent with the high incidence rate, children needing Tier 3 intervention often are those with ADHD. Intervention at this tier is individualized and based on assessment information; it requires significantly more effort than Tier 1 or 2 interventions. Therefore, it is important to first ensure Tiers 1 and 2 interventions have been implemented as designed and that they have been in place a sufficient amount of time to be effective.

Tier 3 intervention is directly linked to assessment information in the form of a functional behavioral assessment. This assessment identifies antecedents or events that precede problem behavior, skill deficits that may contribute to problem behavior, and consequences that may reinforce the problem behavior. This information informs a comprehensive individualized intervention that is assessment derived.

To initiate Tier 3 intervention, the first step is to identify the behavior targeted for change. When a child displays multiple problem behaviors, they need to be prioritized for intervention purposes. Following the guidelines developed by Janney and Snell (2000; see Chapter 3), *destructive* behaviors (e.g., self-injury, aggression) should be the first priority for intervention. Second priority is given to *disruptive* behaviors, or those that interfere with social, emotional, and preacademic development but do not cause an immediate danger (e.g., tantrums, noncompliance). Behavior that is *distracting* is the last priority for intervention. This type of behavior does not result in learning and social delays but may be stigmatizing and age inappropriate (e.g., talking excessively). When prioritizing behaviors for intervention, consensus should be reached among teaching staff, care providers, and family members that the behaviors are important to change and are reasonably prioritized.

Many times a single intervention may reduce more than one problem behavior. This occurs when behaviors fall into the same response class. That is, different forms of a behavior (e.g., aggression, disruption, noncompliance) occur for the same reason or serve the same function (i.e., to escape a difficult task). Thus, it is usually not necessary to develop interventions for every problem behavior. Instead, after an intervention is implemented, an assessment can be conducted to determine the problem behaviors that remain and require additional interventions.

In addition to measuring problem behavior, appropriate behavior should also be measured, particularly behavior that is taught as a replacement for problem behavior. That is, if a child engages in aggression to obtain toys from others, part of his intervention plan will include teaching him to ask for toys in an appropriate way. It is important to measure whether this appropriate behavior is being learned. When children reliably engage in appropriate behavior in situations that previously caused problem behavior, it is likely that problem behavior will be eliminated over the long term.

After target behaviors have been identified and prioritized and appropriate replacement behavior selected, they should be operationally defined so that observers are able to recognize unmistakably whether the behavior occurred. This means that the operational definition describes behavior in a way that can be observed and measured. An example of an operational definition that would be difficult to observe and measure is "fidgeting in class." A better definition that could be observed objectively and measured would be "moving body, legs, or arms for longer than 3 seconds without the purpose of completing a specific task or activity." Similarly, "appropriate interactions" is less specific than "asking a peer if he can join in play using an appropriate tone of voice." Specific operational definitions facilitate communication and allow an objective determination of behavior change.

In addition to defining the target and replacement behavior, a method of recording occurrences of the behavior must be developed (Miltenberger, 2005). Behavior can be measured using the dimension of frequency (i.e., number of occurrences) for brief, discrete behavior (e.g., hitting a peer, throwing a toy); duration (length of occurrence) for behavior that occurs across time (e.g., tantrums, out of seat); intensity (the force of a behavior) when the goal is to modify the behavior's strength (e.g., voice volume); or latency (length of time to initiate behavior) when the objective is to decrease the time from a particular prompt (e.g., instruction to "line up") to initiation of behavior (e.g., child begins to walk toward the line). See Chapter 1 for additional details on measurement systems.

After target behaviors have been identified and defined and a measurement system selected, a functional assessment is conducted. The purpose of a functional assessment is to gather information about events that are associated with problem behavior. This information allows an intervention to be developed that focuses on changing those events identified to be associated with problems. In this way, an intervention is likely to be more effective than one that is randomly selected (Kern, O'Neill, & Starosta, 2005).

Information is collected on *antecedents*, or events that precede the problem behavior. These may include a request to perform a task (e.g., "Hang up your coat," "Clean up your toys"), restricted access to something desirable (e.g., removal of a toy, termination of a preferred activity), or the absence of attention (e.g., paraprofessional is playing with another child and target child is unable to obtain her attention).

Another type of information gathered is *consequences*, or events that follow problem behavior. Typically, preschool teachers, staff, or peers respond in some way when problem behavior occurs. Although usually unintended, the response often functions as reinforcement, thus maintaining the problem behavior. For instance, when a child's tantrum is followed by a teacher's instruction to peers that they must play with her, this would reinforce the tantrum by ensuring that the child obtains the desired activity of play with peers. Consequences function to reinforce behavior either by allowing a child to gain something desirable (positive reinforcement), such as attention or a preferred activity or item, or by allowing a child to escape something undesirable (negative reinforcement), such as a difficult academic demand. In preschool classrooms, adults must divide their attention among many children; hence, a child may engage in problem behavior as a way to get adult attention (positive reinforcement). Also, a characteristic of many young children with ADHD is social difficulties; therefore, they may not have learned how to obtain the attention of others in an appropriate manner. Silly or immature behaviors are common and often reinforced by peer responses, such as turning toward the child and laughing, or adult responses, such as providing corrective statements or reprimands. In this case, the problem behavior is reinforced with peer or adult attention, and behavior is described as serving an attention function. Also, young children with ADHD often lack impulse control or have difficulty waiting their turn and will take items from others or fail to share. In this case, behavior is positively reinforced through access, serving an attention function. Conversely, a variety of tasks can be difficult for young children with ADHD, such as those that require following multiple-step directions, waiting, and sitting or paying attention for periods of time. When problem behaviors occur in these situations, teachers often do not persist with the task requirements, and the child is negatively reinforced, with problem behavior serving an escape function.

It is also important to determine whether a child has *skill deficits* that might be contributing to problem behavior. Problem behavior often occurs because children have not learned the skills necessary to complete tasks successfully, interact appropriately with others, or engage in age-expected play. Further, in preschool settings, young children may experience expectations that have not been required at home, such as sitting still and paying attention during circle time. When children have difficulties due to skill deficits, they often engage in problem behaviors to avoid the demand requirements. Intervention must include teaching new skills or alternative replacement behaviors so that problem behaviors are no longer necessary. For example, Marcia's teacher observed that when she was engaged in activities with her peers, such as sandbox play, she hoarded toys and would not share. For this reason, her peers chose not to engage her in play. By identifying Marcia's particular problem with play (i.e., skill deficit), her intervention plan included teaching her to play with one toy at a time and share the others with her peers (new skill) as well as asking her peers if she could have a turn playing with a toy (replacement behavior).

A final type of information important to intervention is distal events that may contribute indirectly to problem behavior. Referred to as *setting events* (or *establishing operations*), distal events are not immediately proximal to problem behavior but influence the likelihood of problem behavior occurring. More specifically, events of this nature do not directly cause problem behavior but instead make problem behavior more likely in the presence of particular antecedents. For example, a routine instruction that a child normally follows without incident, such as picking up his toys before snack time, may cause problem behaviors when the child is extremely fatigued (setting event). In addition to fatigue, hunger is another common event that plays a role in occurrences of problem behavior among young children. When problem behavior occurs inconsistently in the presence of a particular antecedent, the presence of a setting event or establishing operation should be considered.

The aforementioned information can be gathered through indirect or direct methods. Indirect methods of gathering information are used at times when problem behavior is not occurring, generally through interview. For preschool-age children, interviews are typically conducted with parents, preschool teachers or day care staff, and other care providers who are familiar with children and their target behaviors. Direct methods of gathering information entail some type of direct observation at the time the behavior problem is occurring. The information gathered, whether indirect or direct, should directly contribute to developing an intervention.

A number of structured interviews and direct observation formats for collecting functional assessment data are available commercially (e.g., Bambara & Kern, 2005; O'Neill et al., 1997). Variations in format may be selected on the basis of the individual preference of a teacher or care provider or consultant and the conditions under which data will be collected. For example, some teachers prefer to keep detailed logs, whereas others opt for a checklist format.

Direct and indirect data are collected on a target behavior and its antecedents, consequences, and possible setting events until patterns can be identified, suggesting events that may trigger the behavior problems and responses that may serve as reinforcement. That is, the data are examined to detect patterns within and across methods. For example, direct observation data collected across 5 days indicated that Aaron engaged in 15 tantrums, 12 of which occurred when peers would not let him join in a game (restricted access). Aaron's mother corroborated the problem by stating in a functional assessment interview that he had difficulties getting along with his cousins and other children in the neighborhood. Hence, the cumulated data suggested that Aaron had difficulties with social interactions, particularly joining activities, and tantrums were reinforced by allowing him access to the activity.

It should be kept in mind that behavior can be persistent even when reinforcement is not constant. For example, if a child's noises successfully gain the attention of her peers on average every fourth time, this may be sufficiently reinforcing to the child for noises to continue. Consequently, the function of behavior is not always evident in that reinforcement may be periodic. Rather, the data should suggest a reasonable explanation for problem behavior.

After functional assessment data are collected, they are summarized to formulate hypotheses. Hypothesis statements serve as a link between assessment information and intervention. In their absence, intervention plans often do not bear a relationship to the functional assessment (e.g., Sasso, Conroy, Stichter, & Fox, 2001). Hypothesis statements identify the antecedent, problem behavior, and presumed function. When relevant, they also describe the setting event or establishing operation. An example of a hypothesis statement is, "When Alysa is required to sit longer than 5 minutes [antecedent], she engages in disruption [problem behavior] to escape circle activity [function]." Another example is, "When peers are playing on Aaron's preferred playground equipment [antecedent], he engages in aggression [problem behavior] to gain access to the equipment [function]." When setting events or establishing operations are involved, they are included in the hypothesis statement in the following manner, "When Raul is tired in the afternoon [setting event] and he is told to complete a letter or number identification task [antecedent], he refuses to comply [problem behavior] to escape the task requirement [function]."

The hypothesis statement should directly implicate intervention approaches. Comprehensive intervention plans include multiple components that focus on changing antecedents to problem behavior, teaching new and replacement skills, modifying reinforcing responses to problem behavior, and eliminating or ameliorating setting events or establishing operations. Each of these components is necessary to reduce problem behavior quickly, maintain the reductions in problem behavior over the long term, and avoid inadvertently reinforcing it.

The first component of an intervention plan is antecedent interventions. Antecedent interventions occur in the absence of problem behavior, reducing the likelihood of its occurrence.

This category of interventions focuses on environmental rearrangement. Specifically, events that precede problem behavior are eliminated or modified in some way so that they no longer trigger the problem behavior. For example, if a child is noncompliant when he is given multiple component instructions (i.e., "Put the toys away, wash your hands, get your lunch box, and come to the lunch table"), an antecedent intervention would be to modify the instructions so that only one is given at a time. Another antecedent intervention for a child who has difficulty sitting for 15-minute circle time would be to schedule periodic breaks (e.g., every 5 minutes) to stand up, stretch, and get a drink of water. For children who engage in problem behavior to gain attention, an antecedent intervention would be to provide attention on a scheduled basis (e.g., every 3 minutes). Transitional warnings are an effective antecedent intervention for young children who have difficulty ending a preferred activity (e.g., Boyajian et al., 2001). A warning that the activity will soon end is issued a few minutes before its ending (e.g., "Outdoor play is over in 2 minutes"), then just before the end of the activity (e.g., "Outdoor play ends in 30 seconds"). Similarly, a schedule can be developed so children can predict when activities will occur throughout the day. Timers can facilitate children's adherence to the schedule and understanding of time allocations.

A second group of interventions involves teaching skills or replacement behaviors. This type of intervention includes instruction to remediate skill deficits and to provide children with an alternative and appropriate way of getting their needs met. Instruction should be linked to the function of problem behavior that was identified during the functional assessment. For example, the assessment may have indicated that a child has difficulties in social contexts because he is not able to share and wait his turn during play, a problem common among young children with ADHD. The skills of sharing and waiting can be systematically taught by having pairs of children play with and exchange a toy for increasing lengths of time. Instruction may begin by having one child play with a toy for 15 seconds, then hand it to a peer to play with. The duration of play can be gradually increased until children are exchanging toys after several minutes. An example of teaching a replacement behavior is instructing a child to ask for help during a difficult task or requesting a break during a lengthy task. This can be done by prompting children that they can ask for help or a break before the beginning of the activity and by providing reminders throughout the activity (e.g., "Remember, Eric, if you need help, raise your hand and ask me to help you"). Unlike antecedent interventions, which are generally quick acting, teaching new and replacement skills often takes time. This is particularly true for young children with ADHD, who may be inattentive or impulsive. Instruction should be systematic (e.g., gradually and systematically increase the amount of time a child needs to play independently before receiving attention) and accompanied by frequent prompts and reminders ("Remember to raise your hand and ask for a break if you can't sit any longer").

Intervention plans also need to include ways to respond to problem behavior when it occurs. Behavioral function needs to be considered when developing consequences. Specifically, consequences should not reinforce the problem behavior. For example, if a child engages in problem behavior to escape difficult work, giving a time out from reinforcement as a consequence will reinforce behavior and cause it to continue. Similarly, initiating a discussion of why it is unacceptable to be disruptive in the classroom will be reinforcing to a child whose disruption serves an attention-seeking function.

Consequence interventions also do not need to be highly punitive. Research indicates that harsh punishment may actually result in an increase in problem behaviors (Mayer & Butterworth, 1979). There are many ways to respond to problem behavior that do not inflict pain, cause humiliation, or withhold basic needs (e.g., food). In addition, consequences can sometimes be instructive. For example, prompting and modeling how to share toys offers an instructive consequence for a child when she is not taking turns. Ignoring problem behavior is effective when it is attention seeking. Persisting with a task, while providing encouragement, can decrease escape-maintained problem behavior.

The final component of an intervention plan involves eliminating or ameliorating setting events or establishing operations when they are found to be associated with problem behavior. In some cases, a setting event can be eliminated. For example, scheduling periodic snacks may eliminate problem behavior associated with hunger. In other situations, it may be difficult to eliminate a setting event. An example is a young child who has problems with peers in the early morning and late afternoon as a result of short-acting medication wearing off. Switching the child to a longer acting medication would eliminate the setting event. If, however, changing medications is not possible, an intervention to ameliorate the setting event would be to schedule an independent activity for the child during those problematic times to avoid interactions with peers that cause difficulties.

# EVALUATING PROGRESS

To ascertain whether intervention is effective, target behavior and replacement behavior are measured just before initiating intervention, then periodically following intervention implementation. Ideally, there will be significant reductions in problem behavior and rapid increases in appropriate behavior (Knoster & Kincaid, 2005). When this pattern emerges, the behavior plan can be considered effective, and it is generally sufficient to continue monitoring behavior periodically.

At times, however, reductions in problem behavior and increases in appropriate behavior are observed, but they occur at a slow rate. Teaching young children with ADHD new behaviors and ensuring that they regularly use those behaviors in situations that have historically been problematic often takes time. When behavior change persists, but at a slow rate, it is important to determine whether the rate of behavior change is sufficient. In the case of serious behavior problems, such as aggression, quick reductions may be critical, and the plan may have to be revised. However, some behaviors, such as replacement and alternative skills, take time to learn so that they spontaneously occur during previously problematic situations. Although progress may be slow, absence of the behavior does not put the child or others at risk. As long as steady progress is observed, the plan should be maintained.

When a behavior plan is judged effective, it should continue to be implemented until there is strong evidence that the child regularly exhibits new skills and that problem behaviors have been well reduced or eliminated for an extended period of time (e.g., several months). At that time, staff may consider whether the plan should be faded. It is particularly important to fade plans that have the potential of resulting in stigma for the child (e.g., plan requires the child's removal from typical classroom activities, such as providing frequent breaks) or are labor-intensive to implement. Fading should be gradual and systematic so that changes in the intervention are not readily discernible to the child. For example, a plan that calls for a 1-minute break from preacademic instruction every 5 minutes can be faded by increasing instruction to 5 minutes and 30 seconds, and decreasing the break by 5 seconds. Subsequently, following every 3 to 5 days without child behavior problems, the academic instruction could be increased by 30 seconds and the break decreased by 5 seconds.

At times, an intervention plan results in few or no reductions in problem behavior and minimal increases in replacement or desirable behavior. This can happen for a number of reasons. Occasionally, the events associated with problem behavior (e.g., antecedents, function) were misidentified. The functional assessment and hypotheses should be reevaluated and revised. It may also be that the interventions have not been implemented with fidelity.

The cause of the fidelity lapse should be determined. It may be that additional training is required for teachers to implement the intervention as designed. When teachers have sufficient training and skills but simply forget to implement the intervention, reminders are helpful. For example, a checklist listing intervention components and when they should be implemented can serve as a reminder. Finally, it may be that the intervention does not offer a good contextual fit and teachers are simply unable to implement the intervention given the circumstances of their additional responsibilities. In this situation, additional supports (e.g., staff) may be added or the plan can modified.

## PRESCHOOL-BASED INTERVENTION CASE EXAMPLE

Ms. Caan was a kindergarten teacher with a classroom of 18 students. She was having difficulty with the behavior of her half-day morning class, so she decided to implement tiered intervention. She began with three simple expectations that she believed would address the major problems in her classroom: "Follow directions," "Keep hands and feet to self," and "Say only kind words." Ms. Caan established an incentive system that would allow children to earn up to three checks every 30 minutes for following each of the rules. In addition, consequences were established for not following the rules, consisting of a reminder for the first violation followed by time out from reinforcement for the second. She practiced the rules with the children, including modeling and role playing appropriate and inappropriate behavior, and reviewed the consequences. After the system was in place for 2 weeks, the children's behavior was greatly improved; however, four children in the class continued to have problems, particularly with social interactions. Thus, Ms. Caan implemented a Tier 2 intervention, small-group social skills. She met with the four children three times each week for 10 minutes to work on three skills: using kind words toward peers, taking turns, and using words to express sadness and anger. During groups, Ms. Caan modeled the expected behavior and role played using problematic scenarios she had observed throughout the school day. After several weeks of social skills group, three of the four children's problem behaviors were nearly eliminated. Mikah, however, continued to exhibit problem behaviors, particularly with peers. Consequently, Ms. Caan initiated Tier 3 individualized, assessment-based intervention for Mikah.

Ms. Caan began by identifying and operationally defining Mikah's problem behavior of disruption. She noted that disruption occurred in the form of any of the following: acting silly and in an age-inappropriate manner, yelling, leaving the area he was supposed to be (e.g., lunch table, line), and using materials improperly. Subsequently, Ms. Caan collected ABC (antecedent–behavior–consequence) data across a week, which revealed that Mikah's disruption occurred primarily when he had to wait (see Figure 4.2). Thus, she developed the hypothesis statement "When Mikah is required to wait, he engages in disruptive behavior to escape the wait." Subsequently, she developed an intervention plan with antecedent strategies (decreasing the time he had to wait and providing him alternative activities when a wait was required), teaching alternative skills (waiting appropriately or asking for something to do) and consistent consequences for inappropriate behavior (prompt to

| ABC DATA | | | |
|---|---|---|---|
| Student: Mikah | Teacher: Ms. Caan | | Observation Dates: 1/7–1/10 |
| DATE/TIME | ANTECEDENT | BEHAVIOR | CONSEQUENCE |
| 1/7; 8:00 | At group table, waiting for snack | Out of seat, playing with toys and acting silly | Told to go back to seat |
| 1/7; 10:20 | On playground, wanted tire swing | Yelling at peers who were on swing and in line | Sent back to classroom |
| 1/7; 11:30 | Finished lunch | Left table, crawled under another table and began making animal noises | Aide brought him back to table |
| 1/8; 9:30 | Finished art project | Using paintbrushes as drumsticks | Materials removed |
| 1/9; 10:15 | In line to go outside | Dropped to knees and began crawling on ground | Sent back to seat, required to line up again |
| 1/9; 10:25 | Playing hopscotch | Screamed at peers, calling them cheaters | Time out on playground |
| 1/9; 11:15 | Forgot lunch, teacher getting him a snack | Left seat, trying to take food from other children | Sent back to seat, required to apologize to peers |
| 1/10; 9:00 | Hand raised waiting for help | Making animal sounds at a loud volume | Helped him with his math problem |
| 1/10; 9:35 | Music class-didn't get instrument | Yelling at music teacher | Sent back to classroom |
| 1/10; | In seat waiting for teacher to start video | Swept items off desk, fell to floor and crawled around | Sent to time out |

Figure 4.2. ABC (antecedent–behavior–consequence) data for Mikah.

### TABLE 4.1
#### Mikah's Kindergarten Behavior Support Plan

| Antecedent interventions | Skill instruction | Consequences |
| --- | --- | --- |
| Hypothesis 1: When Mikah is required to wait, he engages in disruptive behavior to escape the wait. | | |
| Organize school day so wait time is minimized.<br>Provide an alternative activity (e.g., small toy that can be kept in pocket) for Mikah to play with when he has to wait. | When wait time is necessary (e.g., after lunch), systematically teach Mikah to tolerate waiting by having him initially wait 30 seconds (then allow him to leave table), then gradually increasing wait by 10 seconds every 3 days; after he tolerates a 3-minute wait, replicate on the playground.<br>Teach Mikah to ask for something else to do when he has to wait. | When disruptive behavior occurs, remind Mikah to wait quietly or ask for something to do; if he leaves his area, ask him to return and then provide reminder. |

wait quietly or ask for something to do, return to seat). These interventions decreased the aversiveness of waiting, systematically increased his tolerance for waiting and taught him an appropriate alternative behavior, and ensured that the consequence did not allow him to escape waiting. Mikah's intervention plan is shown in Table 4.1. Teacher-collected data revealed a gradual decline in problem behavior, and within 3 months, Mikah seldom exhibited disruption.

## CONCLUSION

Recent models of intervention delivery in preschool (and school) settings have emphasized a tiered approach. Such an approach has proved highly effective because it is based on a prevention premise in which *all* children receive instruction in appropriate behavior, taught through classwide or programwide expectations. This Tier 1 intervention will eliminate the behavior problems of the majority of children in a given classroom. However, for the small number of students who are nonresponders to Tier 1 intervention, Tier 2 intervention provides additional support, such as small-group instruction in a particular skill area (e.g., sharing). For young children with or at risk for ADHD who exhibit significant symptoms, Tier 3 intervention may be

*Issue: My colleague believes that ADHD is a biological disorder and it is impossible for children with ADHD to control their behavior.*

Potential solution: Regardless of the cause of ADHD, an extensive amount of research has shown that children with ADHD can be taught to reduce problem behavior and engage in appropriate behavior. A reluctant colleague might be convinced by data that illustrate behavior change.

*Issue: I am concerned that we do not have the expertise in our preschool to conduct a functional behavioral assessment.*

Potential solution: The behavior of young children is generally far less complex than that of older children, and it is often quite easy to identify behavioral function. In fact, research has demonstrated that observers with little formal training (e.g., paraeducators) are able to collect accurate data to identify the events that precede and follow problem behavior. It is also advisable to use a team approach so that educators with different types of expertise can work together and help one another complete the functional assessment process.

*Issue: Teachers in our preschool do not believe in reinforcing children. They claim it will make children dependent on adults to feel good about themselves.*

Potential solution: It is the responsibility of adults to teach children to behave appropriately. Too often, adults rely only on punishment (e.g., time out) when children misbehave and do not recognize when children behave appropriately. This is particularly devastating for children who seek attention, regardless of the form. That is, they learn that they are able to obtain attention by engaging in undesirable behavior. Praise and reinforcement have been demonstrated to improve appropriate behavior and decrease inappropriate behavior in numerous studies across decades of research. Further, an environment characterized by predominantly positive adult–child interactions is much more pleasant for both adults and children.

necessary. Intervention at this level is linked to the results of a functional behavioral assessment and involves a multicomponent plan, including preventive strategies, skill instruction, and appropriate consequences.

There are challenges that may be encountered when implementing the approach described in this chapter. Common challenges and potential solutions are described in Exhibit 4.1

# 5

# PROMOTION OF ACADEMIC SKILLS

As previous chapters have indicated, young children with attention-deficit/hyperactivity disorder (ADHD) are at higher than average risk for exhibiting deficits in reading, mathematics, and language skills. Upon entry into kindergarten, children with this disorder are likely to be behind their typically developing classmates in basic math concepts and prereading skills (Lahey et al., 1998; Mariani & Barkley, 1997; Shelton et al., 1998). For example, DuPaul, McGoey, Eckert, and VanBrakle (2001) found that a sample of 58 preschool-age children with ADHD scored on average approximately 1 standard deviation below a sample of 36 typically developing peers on a test of cognitive development and preacademic skills (i.e., the Battelle Developmental Inventory; Newborg, Stock, & Wnek, 1988). Specifically, 3- to 5-year-old children with ADHD scored significantly lower than control participants with respect to perceptual discrimination, memory, reasoning, and conceptual development skills (see Figure 5.1). This is particularly concerning given the strong relationship between early skills and later achievement (e.g., Storch & Whitehurst, 2002). That is, children who lack early literacy and numeracy skills tend to score behind their peers academically in elementary school and beyond. The fact that young children with ADHD are at significant risk for academic impairment over the long term is supported by data indicating

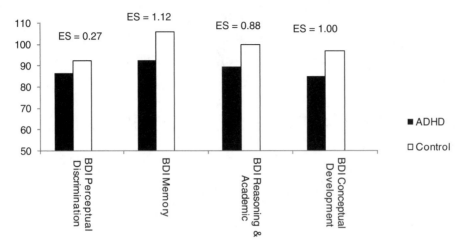

*Figure 5.1.* Standard scores on the Battelle Developmental Inventory (BDI) for young children with attention-deficit/hyperactivity disorder (ADHD) and typically developing controls. Data are from DuPaul, McGoey, Eckert, and VanBrakle (2001). ES = effect size.

that children with this disorder are significantly more likely to be placed in special education programs during the early elementary school years (Lahey et al., 1998); are likely to underachieve in reading, math, and spelling (Massetti et al., 2008); and are less likely to complete high school than their typically developing peers (Barkley, Murphy, & Fischer, 2008).

The results of an investigation conducted by O'Reilly (2002) underscore the degree to which young children with ADHD enter elementary school trailing behind their typically developing classmates in critical areas of academic functioning. The trajectory of prereading and reading skills was examined in a small sample of kindergartners and first graders exhibiting significant ADHD symptoms and a matched sample of comparison children. The Dynamic Indicators of Basic Early Literacy Skills (DIBELS; Kaminski & Good, 1996) was used to assess acquisition of skills over three time points (fall, winter, and spring) during the school year. Kindergarten children with ADHD differed from the comparison sample by approximately 0.5 standard deviations in early literacy skills at all three assessment points. Similar group differences in terms of oral reading fluency were found for first graders in this study. Further, the first graders with ADHD symptoms exhibited a slower growth rate in oral reading fluency relative to an at-risk comparison group and also scored below the 50th percentile using local district DIBELS norms (see Figure 5.2 for fall and winter data). Thus, many young children with ADHD enter elementary

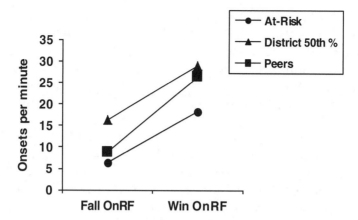

*Figure 5.2.* Mean onset recognition fluency (OnRF) scores for kindergarten at-risk and comparison peer groups compared with 50th percentile on district norms for fall and winter (Win) benchmarks. From *Early Literacy Skill Development of Kindergartners and First-Graders At-Risk for Externalizing Behavior Disorders,* by M. O'Reilly, 2002, unpublished manuscript, University of Massachusetts Amherst. Reprinted by permission of the author.

school behind their classmates in critical academic skills, and this deficit continues through the early elementary grades and beyond (Massetti et al., 2008).

Early academic skills intervention is critically important given the association of academic impairments with ADHD and the fact that these children enter elementary school already behind typically developing classmates. The purpose of this chapter is to describe intervention strategies that can be implemented in home and preschool settings to enhance the development of language, reading, and math skills. Because few studies have evaluated strategies specifically in the ADHD population, interventions that have been used with other at risk groups (e.g., children with behavior problems in general, children from socially disadvantaged backgrounds, children at risk for academic failure) are included. Features that may enhance early intervention for the ADHD population are highlighted. Future directions for research in this area are delineated, with an emphasis on developing strategies that are feasible and effective for implementation in real-world settings.

## STRATEGIES TO PROMOTE EARLY LANGUAGE SKILLS

The development of early language skills (e.g., word recognition, vocabulary) is critical to cognitive growth, school readiness, and reading. Although children's cognitive abilities have an impact on early language development, it is clear that home and preschool environments play an important role as well. For example, Hart and Risley (1995) found that children's vocabulary development was directly and strongly related to language exposure in the home setting. Further, this exposure was correlated with socioeconomic status: Children from poor families exhibited significantly limited vocabularies relative to children from middle- and upper-class backgrounds, primarily as a result of limited language exposure rather than income per se. Thus, strategies to enhance vocabulary growth and related language skills in young children should be used for at risk populations, including those with ADHD. Specific approaches to promoting early language skill development include behavioral strategies to prompt and reinforce targeted skills (e.g., blended communication and behavior support [BCBS]; Hancock, Kaiser, & Delaney, 2002), social communication skills training (Craig-Unkefer & Kaiser, 2002), enhanced milieu teaching (Alpert & Kaiser, 1992), and strategies focused on narrative and vocabulary skills (Peterson, Jesso, & McCabe, 1999).

Behavioral strategies can be used to promote children's communication behaviors and language production. Hancock et al. (2002) described a parent-implemented BCBS system for use with children who are at risk for language and behavior difficulties. Parent educators work individually with parents to promote parent responsiveness to children's verbal behavior, use of contingent praise to promote child compliance, and other parental strategies to promote children's use of language (see Table 5.1). Each 30- to 45-minute training session includes 10 to 15 minutes to provide parents with feedback about previous sessions (e.g., correct use of strategies), with the remainder of the time focused on introducing new skills and information. Strategies for each session are taught using verbal instruction, written handouts, role plays, and videotapes. Further, parents are given specific instructions on how to use the strategy during play with their child in the clinic or preschool setting while the parent educator observes. Parent educators also model procedures with children and coach parents as they attempt to use the strategies with their children. Feedback is provided following each session. Training continues until parent behavior reaches criterion performance (see Table 5.1) or until 30 training sessions take place. Hancock et al. examined BCBS effects for five young children with language delays and behavior difficulties from low socioeconomic backgrounds. Following training, parent behavior met criterion performance levels for use of BCBS strategies and the changes in parental behaviors generalized to the home setting and were maintained 6 months after intervention. As a result, children showed improvements in behavior and language, but generalization and maintenance of these changes varied across children.

Another parent-mediated intervention approach involves strategies designed to enhance children's narrative skills (Peterson, Jesso, & McCabe, 1999). First, parents are provided with information regarding the types of

## TABLE 5.1
Blended Communication and Behavior Support Intervention Goals,
Rationale, Measures, and Criteria for Parent Behavior

| Goal | Rationale | Measure | Criterion |
|---|---|---|---|
| Balance turns | Create a conversational framework for interaction | Discrepancy of turns (based on no. parent verbal turns minus no. child verbal and nonverbal turns) | 0 |
| Give children opportunity to respond | Encourage child-initiated utterances | No. parent pause errors (i.e., two or more consecutive parent utterances without a 3-second pause for child to respond) | < 5 |
| Increase parent responsiveness to child verbal behavior | Meaningful, related responses encourage child communication and provide context-specific language models | % of child verbalizations followed by responsive feedback | > 80% |
| Give simple, clear instructions | Children respond best if instruction is at their language level and requests only one response | No. and % of correct parent command episodes during transitions | > 80% |
| Decrease frequency of instructions during play | Giving commands only for "important" behaviors will increase child compliance | No. parent commands during play | < 5 |
| Increase positive responses following child compliance | Differentiate consequences for compliance and noncompliance to increase child compliance | % of child's compliant behaviors to which parents appropriately responded | > 80% |
| Increase corrective responses following child noncompliance | Differentiate consequences for compliance and noncompliance to increase child compliance | % of child's non-compliant behaviors to which parents appropriately responded | > 80% |
| Decrease parent negative verbal behavior | Negative behavior by parent models negative behavior for child and creates negative affect in interaction | No. parent negative statements | 0 |
| Increase parent praise | Children learn from positive consequences and praise makes interactions affectively more positive | No. parent praise statements | > 10 |
| Provide models of appropriate language | New language forms are learned through modeling | % of expansions of child utterances at target level | > 30% |

narrative interactions that can foster children's language development. Next, parent interaction styles that could enhance narrative skills necessary for school success are promoted by emphasizing parental behaviors that prompt and reinforce developing language (see Exhibit 5.1). Parents are shown transcripts and listen to audiotapes of mothers employing these narrative elicitation strategies with their children. Role play and feedback are then used to encourage parent practice of these strategies. Treatment sessions occur bimonthly over the course of 1 year, with interim telephone calls to promote ongoing use of the strategies. Peterson et al. (1999) found that young children from economically disadvantaged backgrounds whose mothers used this approach demonstrated significant vocabulary development and improvement in narrative abilities relative to a control group.

Milieu strategies can also be used to promote increased verbal behavior in at-risk preschool children. Craig-Unkefer and Kaiser (2002) used a three-component social communication training program to promote more frequent and complex verbal interactions among six preschool children at risk for language delays and behavior problems (see Table 5.2). Children are divided into dyads and participate in 20-minute intervention sessions three or four times per week. The first part of each session is an advanced play organizer in which an interventionist works with the dyad to choose a play theme (e.g., grocery store) and label toys that might be used for play in the context of the chosen theme. Next, dyads play with each other while the interventionist prompts and reinforces appropriate verbal and play behavior, as necessary. Following each play session, a review time is used to promote children's discussion of what they played with, how they played with the toys, and whether they enjoyed the play interaction. This intervention led to an increase in the number of social communication behaviors exhibited by each child during play and also enhanced the complexity and diversity of verbal utterances.

EXHIBIT 5.1
Parent Strategies for Enhancing Children's Narrative Skills

1. Talk with your child frequently and consistently about past experiences.
2. Spend a lot of time talking about each topic.
3. Ask plenty of "wh" questions and few "yes/no" questions. As part of this, ask questions about the context or setting of the events, especially where and when they took place.
4. Listen carefully to what your child is saying, and encourage elaboration.
5. Encourage your child to say more than one sentence at a time by using back channel responses or repeating what your child has just said.
6. Follow your child's lead. Talk about what your child wants to talk about.

From "Encouraging Narratives in Preschoolers: An Intervention Study" by C. Peterson, B. Jesso, and A. McCabe, 1999, *Journal of Child Language, 26,* p. 53. Copyright 1999 by Cambridge University Press. Adapted with permission.

## STRATEGIES TO PROMOTE EARLY READING SKILLS

Given the importance of reading for short- and long-term academic achievement, many early intervention approaches have been developed to enhance skills fundamental to reading development. We have incorporated strategies to promote early literacy into our early intervention for ADHD protocol. More intensive early reading intervention strategies have included shared book reading (Justice, Kaderavek, Xitao, Sofka, & Hunt, 2009), phonological awareness training (Koutsoftas, Harmon, & Gray, 2009), explicit emergent literacy intervention (Justice, Chow, Capellini, Flanigan, & Colton, 2003), and computer-assisted instruction for phonological sensitivity (Lonigan et al., 2003).

The early intervention for ADHD protocol described in Chapter 2 includes parent- and teacher-led activities designed to enhance early reading skills. Specifically, one parent education session during Tier 1 group-based intervention is devoted to development of early literacy skills (see Chapter 3). The primary curriculum guide used to create early literary experiences is *Assessment and Training of Pre-academic Skills: Home*. A teacher version, *Ladders to Literacy: A Preschool Activity Book* (Notari-Syverson, O'Connor, & Vadasy, 1998), can be used in preschool settings. The program offers multiple activity choices and opportunities for practice, thus making it appropriate for children at a variety of developmental levels. Activities and experiences contained in *Ladders to Literacy* fall into three broad areas that have been identified to influence children's literacy development, including print and book awareness, meta-linguistic awareness, and oral language.

*Ladders to Literacy* contains simple activities designed to be feasible for parents and can be completed in the context of other activities (e.g., while washing the dishes or driving the car). Parents are provided activity descriptions on index cards for easy access and are instructed to complete at least one activity daily, lasting approximately 15 to 20 minutes. An example of an activity is parents ask children to predict what will happen next when reading a familiar story.

Home-based literacy activities are supplemented with preschool strategies designed to enhance reading skills. As much as possible, these strategies are designed to meet individual needs based on assessment data. For example, phonemic segmentation fluency, letter naming fluency, and picture naming fluency can be assessed using the Dynamic Indicators of Basic Early Literacy Skills (DIBELS; Kaminski & Good, 1996). These data can help teachers individualize instruction on an ongoing basis.

The Ladders to Literacy program is used as the instructional intervention because it contains an extensive curriculum for early childhood teachers. Each activity is used to teach or reinforce a specific skill (e.g., awareness of sounds). Activities are categorized into three levels of task demand: high demand–low support, medium demand–medium support, and low demand–high support. These correspond to the demand of the task on the child and the level of adult assistance needed to complete the activity. This system of categorization facilitates selection and scheduling of tasks depending on child characteristics and ongoing demands on the teacher. In addition, tasks contain multiple skills or goals, along with adaptations for children with disabilities (e.g., hearing, motor, or visual impairments). Thus, they are suitable for children with diverse learning needs.

The specific effects of the literacy skills component of our early intervention protocol are difficult to discern given that these strategies are delivered in the context of a larger intervention. However, it is important to note that the trajectory of DIBELS scores over a 2-year period for children receiving early intervention was significantly positive, presumably because of the literacy skills intervention component (DuPaul, Kern, et al., 2009). Nevertheless, more intensive strategies to promote early reading skills may be necessary, especially for those children who do not show growth in early literacy skills in response to the Ladders to Literacy activities.

## Shared Book Reading

One of the simplest, yet most effective, methods for building early reading skills is for parents and other adults to read books to children. In fact, shared book reading, without directly targeting oral language abilities, has been found to improve children's vocabulary, grammar skills, and letter-sound awareness (van Kleeck, 2008). The value of shared book reading is further enhanced when adults and children discuss story content in an interactive way. This is sometimes referred to as *dialogic reading* (Zevenbergen & Whitehurst, 2003). With interactive dialogue, shared book reading can address both decoding and comprehension skills. Comprehension skills are directly targeted by having adults ask literal and inferential questions about stories (see Table 5.3) and embedding scripted questions in storybooks before sharing them. Scripted questions are particularly important for adults who are less comfortable or experienced in reading to children and can structure the interaction to best address comprehension skills. Family literacy workshops can be used to encourage parents to engage in effective book-sharing techniques. In fact, Primavera (2000) found that book-sharing workshops led to significant increases in parents of low-income preschoolers reading to their children, as well as significant enhancement of children's language skills and interest in reading. Similar findings were obtained for a sample of Head Start preschoolers with language impairments exposed to book sharing with embedded questions intervention twice per week over 8 weeks (van Kleeck, Vander

TABLE 5.2
Social Communication Training: Intervention Components and Activities

| Intervention component | Interventionist activities |
|---|---|
| Advanced play organization | 1. Interventionist announces play theme for session. |
| | 2. Interventionist labels toys to be used in play session. |
| | 3. Interventionist provides at least one play option for child dyad. |
| | 4. Interventionist allows children to suggest at least one play option. |
| | 5. Interventionist prompts children to play and talk to each other during session. |
| Play session | 1. Play area is set up to allow easy access to play materials. |
| | 2. Interventionist uses verbal redirects (models, direct instructions or indirect instructions) and reflective statements to sustain children's play interaction. |
| Review session | 1. Interventionist asks children what types of play interaction occurred. |
| | 2. Interventionist asks children whether they enjoyed playing with their partner. |

From "Improving the Social Communication Skills of At-Risk Preschool Children in a Play Context" by L. A. Craig-Unkefer and A. P. Kaiser, 2002, *Topics in Early Childhood Special Education, 22,* p. 8. Copyright 2002 by Sage Publications Inc. Adapted with permission.

Woude, & Hammett, 2006). In fact, moderate to large effect sizes in literal and inferential comprehension skills were found between the intervention and control groups in this study.

Shared book reading is an example of an activity that would occur in home and preschool settings that encourage literacy (i.e., literacy environments). Parent involvement in early literacy activities with their children may be associated with long-term progress in reading achievement (Drouin, 2009). The creation of literacy environments in preschool classrooms is also strongly encouraged by various early childhood education organizations (e.g., National Association of Education for Young Children). Unfortunately, the majority of center-based child-care and preschool programs do not engage in recommended literacy promoting activities, at least not at levels that are considered effective for enhancing early reading skill development (Dunn, Beach, & Kontos, 2000). Thus, children at risk for early reading failure, including those with ADHD, will require additional intervention, particularly if their homes and/or preschools are not literacy-promoting environments.

**Phonological Awareness Training**

Phonological awareness (i.e., ability to distinguish speech sounds separately from their meaning) is a critical precursor to decoding and reading readiness (Beck & Juel, 1999). Phonemic awareness (i.e., recognition of and ability to manipulate individual phonemes in words) is a subcomponent of phonological awareness and the strongest predictor of reading decoding (Hulme et al., 2002). Thus, phonemic awareness training is considered an important strategy for enhancing early reading skills in at-risk populations. Explicit instruction in phonemic awareness includes teaching children to listen for specific letter sounds in the environment; enhancing conceptual understanding of phonemes using manipulatives (e.g., toys), letters, and letter sounds; and asking children to combine the concepts of sound and phoneme location in words that are being taught in their preschool classrooms (Koutsoftas, Harmon, & Gray, 2009).

Koutsoftas et al. (2009) examined the effects of phonemic awareness training as a Tier 2 intervention for 34 young children who were at risk for early reading failure based on minimal response to Tier 1 phonological awareness training in their preschool classrooms. Intervention scripts were designed to meet phonemic awareness objectives using direct instruction components including teaching objective, anticipatory set, purpose, input, modeling, checking for understanding, guided practice, and closure (see Table 5.4 for a sample script). Twelve 20- to 25-minute training sessions were conducted over several weeks with small groups of children in the classroom setting. More than 70% of the participating children showed moderate to large improvements in phonemic awareness skills as a function of training. Similar positive outcomes for at-risk preschoolers have been obtained for explicit emergent literacy intervention (i.e., name writing, alphabet recognition, and phonological awareness activities; Justice et al., 2003) and computer-assisted instruction in phonological sensitivity (Lonigan et al., 2003).

Although these early reading skill strategies have established efficacy with various at-risk populations (e.g., children from low-income families, children with language skill delays), it is important to note that these interventions have not been evaluated with the ADHD population. There is at least one study that shows limited effects of Tier 1 phonological awareness training on the reading outcomes of preschool children exhibiting challenging behaviors. Elliot, Prior, Merrigan, and Ballinger (2002) randomly assigned a sample of preschoolers with behavior difficulties to one of four groups: (a) phonological skills prereading training alone, (b) parent training in behavior management alone, (c) combined prereading and parent training, or (d) no-treatment control. Children's behavior and reading skills were assessed at baseline, immediately following treatment, and at 1- and 2-year follow-up periods. Significant improvements in behavior were obtained for the two groups receiving parent training; however, the prereading intervention was not associated with improvements in reading skills. Elliot et al. (2002) concluded that preschoolers with significant behavior difficulties may require

TABLE 5.3
Shared Storybook Reading:
Examples of Questions in Relation to Story Elements

| Story element | Example of literal or inferential question |
|---|---|
| Initiating event/problem | What is the main character's big problem/desire? What is this story about? |
| Internal response | How do you think the main character feels? What do you think the main character might be thinking? Why do you think so? |
| Goal/theme | What does the main character want to happen/want to get? What was the main character trying to do all the way through this story? |
| Attempts | What did the main character do? What happened here? What do you think will happen next? Why? Do you think it will work? |
| Consequences of individual attempts and internal response | Did the attempt work? What do you think the main character is thinking/feeling here? |
| Solution/outcome | Did the main character get what he or she wanted? What was it? |
| Location | Where does this story happen? |
| Time, duration | What time of the day/year is it? |
| Characters | Who is this story about? Who is in this story? |
| World knowledge | What do you already know about this? |
| Using context of story to define words | What do you think this word means? Why? |
| Judgments of morality, convention, or anomaly | Was that a good thing to do? Is that what we usually do? |

From "Preschool Foundations for Later Reading Comprehension: Importance of and Ideas for Targeting Inferencing in Storybook-sharing Interventions" by A. Van Kleeck, 2008, *Psychology in the Schools, 45,* p. 633. Copyright 2008 by John Wiley and Sons. Adapted with permission.

more intensive prereading interventions carried out over longer periods for reading success to occur.

## STRATEGIES TO PROMOTE EARLY MATHEMATICS SKILLS

Comparatively little research has examined specific early intervention strategies for the development of mathematics skills. Thus, recommended approaches have limited empirical support. The Number Worlds program (Griffin, 2007) is a promising intervention protocol addressing early mathematics skills through direct instruction from pre-kindergarten through sixth grade. Mathematics is viewed as comprising three "worlds": the world of real quantities that exist in space and time, the world of counting numbers and iconic symbols (e.g., spoken language), and the world of formal symbols such as written numerals and operation signs. Number Worlds leads children through a developmental sequence that is consistent with the putative natural progression of math knowledge.

Five key teaching strategies are used in the Number Worlds program (Griffin, 2007). First, for each math concept taught, instruction begins in the world of real quantities (i.e., using concrete objects and examples). Instruction remains in this "world" until children demonstrate understanding of the quantities or quantity transformations that underlie the specific concept. Second, children are provided with sufficient opportunity to use oral language to process concepts covered in the world of real quantities to make sense of this information. Instruction remains in the world of counting numbers long enough for children to demonstrate their understanding of a particular concept. Third, the world of formal symbols is gradually and systematically introduced by using familiar contexts and concepts. Fourth, the selection of math concepts for instruction is based on children's current level of understanding following a natural developmental progression. Finally, children should be encouraged to use natural strategies for solving math problems while introducing novel problem-solving strategies so that they have several effective choices. The Number Worlds program has been evaluated longitudinally with several samples of children. Significant improvements in various math skills (e.g., number knowledge, computational skills) have been found for children receiving instruction in the Number Worlds program relative to control participants (Griffin, 2007).

Our early intervention protocol takes a similar approach to the Number Worlds program in promoting early numeracy skills. One session of Tier 1 group-based parent education is devoted to promoting numeracy skills (see Chapter 3). As is the case for early reading skills, parents are urged to take an active approach to incorporating numeracy learning into everyday activities. Further, activities require children to manipulate objects in real-world tasks to make math concepts as concrete as possible. The primary objective of home-based activities is for children to develop a number sense. A child who has a well-developed number sense (a) is able to think about numbers in a variety of ways, (b) has a sense of what numbers mean, (c) is able to make comparisons, and (d) has the ability to perform mental math. Nine related number sense skills are addressed: rote counting, quantity concepts, counting using one-to-one correspondence, representations, number identification, number naming, number writing, adding and subtracting, and fractions.

For each number sense skill, parents are provided with an operational description of the skill as well as a variety of activities that can promote it. *Rote counting* involves children starting at the number 1 and saying numbers in sequence without the use of objects. Possible activities include counting songs, playing the "how high we can count" game, and jumping game ("1, 2, 3, up we go"). Children should also understand the *quantity concepts* of more, less, most, and least. These concepts can be taught in the context of meal-time portion comparison (e.g., "Who has more peas on their plate?") or when playing with toys (e.g., "Who has the least number of blocks?"). *Counting using one-to-one correspondence* involves counting objects one at a time. This skill can be taught while setting the table, handing out cookies, or putting away toys. A critical number sense skill is for children to be able to recognize that numbers represent a specific quantity of objects. Thus, *representation* involves children being able to show the correct number of objects to match a given number. Activities to practice this skill can be incorporated into cooking ("Please give me three spoonfuls of sugar") or playing tea party (e.g., "Can I have two cookies, please?"). *Number identification* involves pointing to a stated number when presented with an array of numbers (e.g., given the numbers 1, 4, and 8, children are asked to point to 4, and they point to the correct number). Activities can include pointing to stated numbers in addresses or on signs when driving or walking. *Number naming* involves saying the correct number name when presented with a number. Activities can include showing a price when in a store (e.g., "How many dollars is this toy?") or playing a memory card game with numbers. In similar fashion, *number writing* is when children write the correct number when asked to do so. Children can help make grocery lists that require numbers, tracing numbers in a coloring book, or writing numbers during play (e.g., in shaving cream).

Two of the nine number sense skills involve more advanced, abstract concepts. *Adding and subtracting* involves presenting children with objects, pictures, or numbers and asking them to find how many there are "all together" (i.e., summing the number of objects) or how many are "left over" (i.e., subtracting one number from another number). Cooking is an ideal activity for teaching these concepts because children can be asked to add or subtract ingredients (e.g., "I'm putting one cup of sugar in the bowl, and when you put one more cup of sugar in, how many cups of sugar will be in the bowl?"; "I put one cup of milk in the bowl, how many more do I need to make two?"). Mealtimes can also lend themselves to practicing addition and subtraction (e.g., "I have five cookies. If I eat two cookies, how many will I have left?"). Finally, young children can learn *fractions*, in which they understand the concepts of "part" and "whole" as well as half and quarter. Possible learning activities include talking about sharing some food (e.g., "Can I have one fourth of the candy bar?") or playing blocks (e.g., "Can I have half of the blocks?").

The final portion of the parent education session involves parents pairing up to generate ideas of possible activities for each math concept and then sharing these ideas with the larger group. Parents are given a homework assignment to write down four ways that they will teach number sense skills to their children before the next parent education session. They are also asked to note how these activities worked so that they can report back to the group at the beginning of the next session.

## ASSESSMENT OF LEARNING OUTCOMES

Learning outcomes can be measured from the perspective of three approaches: critical skills mastery, general outcomes, and responsiveness to intervention (Hoskyn, 2009). Each of these approaches has its strengths and weaknesses, and thus measurement choice depends on the goals for assessment. Ideally, measurement will be conducted using more than one approach in order to obtain a comprehensive picture of children's academic status.

The critical skills mastery approach is based on the assumption that children's specific skills are connected such that growth occurs in the context of a developmental hierarchy (Phaneuf & Silberglitt, 2003). Thus, certain basic skills (e.g., letter recognition) must be present before more advanced skills (e.g., recognition of phonemes) can develop. This approach to assessment is used to identify specific reading or math skills that are present and absent in a child's repertoire so that interventions can target skill development in a hierarchical fashion. Thus, a skills mastery assessment approach is critical for the development of effective and efficient skills instruction strategies.

The general outcomes approach to assessment relies on curriculum-based measures or more distal indices (e.g., memory or general language abilities) of skills development (Shapiro, 2004). Curriculum-based measures require children to complete brief probes of reading or math skills taken directly from the curriculum that is being taught (Shinn, 1998). General outcomes in areas that are related to academic skill development may also be assessed, including memory, language, and school readiness. For example, the Bracken Basic Concept Scale—Revised (Bracken, 1998) provides general outcomes for various areas of school readiness, including basic literacy and numeracy skills. The primary goal of this assessment approach is to characterize children's overall status with respect to reading and math skills as well as related areas of cognitive development at a specific point in time. Measures can be collected before and after intervention to document whether instructional strategies have made a difference at a global level.

The responsiveness to intervention assessment approach is used to evaluate children's rate of academic skill development as a function of instructional intervention (Jimerson, Burns, & VanDerHeyden, 2007). This assessment strategy involves repeated measurement of situational and curriculum-based learning before, during, and after instructional changes. The degree to which an intervention is helpful is determined by examining change in the trajectory or slope of academic skills growth over time. Thus, this assessment approach can be used to determine whether a specific intervention is effective or whether changes to instruction are necessary (e.g., if slope change does not meet a target goal).

## IMPORTANT FEATURES OF STRATEGIES
## TO PROMOTE EARLY ACADEMIC SKILLS

Effective strategies for promoting the development of early academic skills share several features that are critical to success. Although most of these interventions have not been specifically evaluated for young children with ADHD, incorporating these features may be especially important in eliciting optimal levels of attention and engagement in this population. Key features include incorporating structured activities into regular routines, making learning fun, implementing interventions that involve both parents and teachers, and using a variety of outcome measures to gauge children's response to intervention (Hoskyn, 2009).

Effective academic strategies for young children often involve taking advantage of incidental learning opportunities. Specifically, learning activities are incorporated into regular routines (e.g., getting dressed in the morning, preparing for meals, driving to school) at home and in the preschool classroom. Parents and teachers can optimize learning opportunities by anticipating these daily routines and proactively structuring learning activities to occur during those times. Thus, rather than waiting for a situation to occur before initiating a learning activity, parents and teachers should plan activities that can be incorporated a priori into a given situation. The Ladders to Literacy program described earlier in this chapter provides many ideas for activities that can be used during many daily routines. The assumption is that children will be more engaged in learning activities that are delivered in the context of a natural situation rather than trying to teach a concept in the abstract. Implementing learning activities in real-world situations may also promote generalization and maintenance of skill development.

For preschoolers, play is a major age-appropriate activity across home and classroom settings. Children at this age are naturally engaged in any interactions that involve play and enjoyment. Thus, learning activities should be presented in playful and enjoyable contexts to maximize children's engagement. This is especially important for capturing the attention of children with ADHD, who are prone to disengage from events that are lengthy and devoid of enjoyment. For example, the phonemic awareness intervention script described in Table 5.4 includes the use of stuffed animals and puppets to playfully engage children in learning initial letter sounds.

## TABLE 5.4
## Sample Intervention Script for Phonemic Awareness Training

| Teaching component | Scripted implementation |
| --- | --- |
| Set/hook | "Remember my friends?" [Show stuffed animal and puppet.] "This is Sammy [show puppet]. "The first sound in Sammy's name is /s/. Sammy's name begins with /s/. This is Maggie [show stuffed animal], the first sound in Maggie's name is /m/. Maggie's name begins with the sound /m/." |
| Purpose | "It is important to listen to names, especially the first sound in names." |
| Input | "We know that the first sound in Sammy's name is /s/, and that the first sound in Maggie's name is /m/. [Show the picture of Superman.] "Do you know who this is? This is Superman, the first sound in his name is /s/." [Show picture of Percy the Train.] "This is Percy. The first sound in his name is /p/." |
| Modeling | "Okay, Sammy [to the puppet], help me out, whose name has the first sound /s/?" [Sammy thinks and then points to Superman.] "Yes, Superman begins with /s/. Nice job, Sammy. Whose name begins with /p/?" [Sammy points to Percy.] "That's right again, Sammy. Percy's name begins with the sound /p/. Wow, Sammy, you really know how to listen for the first sound in someone's name." |
| Checking for understanding | 1. "Now, let's see how well you children can listen for these characters' names." [Have all pictures facing the children. Each child should get at least two turns identifying the pictures.] "Whose name begins with /m/, /d/, /p/, /s/, /t/, /b/?" [Reinforce all correct responses. Provide correct responses for erred responses.]<br>2. "Okay, now I am really going to see if you are listening carefully. Raise your hand if I say the first sound in your name." [Say each child's name by saying just the initial sound in the name.] |
| Guided practice | [Have each child take a turn identifying other children by the first sound in their name. You can have one child stand next to you and ask them to say another child's name but just use the first sound of their name. This can be done by having the children say, "Raise your hand . . . (First sound of child's name goes here)." or "Stand up . . . (First sound of child's name goes here).")] |
| Closure | "Today we learned about listening for the first sound in someone's name, and wow, you all did a good job. Thank you everyone for working so hard." [Ask the children to line up by saying just the first sound in their name.] |

*Note.* Materials: Stuffed animal, puppet, pictures of Superman, Bert, Donald Duck, Mickey Mouse, Thomas the Train, and Percy the Train. Teaching Objective: Children will identify the names of classmates and familiar fictional characters when given the initial sound only. From "The Effect of Tier 2 Intervention for Phonemic Awareness in a Response-to-Intervention Model in Low-Income Preschool Classrooms," by A. D. Koutsoftas, M. T. Harmon, and S. Gray, 2009, *Language, Speech, and Hearing Services in Schools, 40,* p. 129. Copyright 2009 by the American Speech–Language–Hearing Association. Adapted with permission.

Intervention approaches that involve parents and teachers working together or at least using similar strategies appear to be more effective over the long term than treatment that is implemented solely by parents or teachers (Hoskyn, 2009). The consistent use of strategies across settings can promote the generalization of skill development and also enhance the collaborative relationship between parents and teachers. Cross-situational consistency and collaboration is especially important when working with children who have a chronic, pervasive disorder like ADHD. For children who are difficult to engage, it is critical to take advantage of every learning opportunity, no matter the setting or situation. Thus, having parents and teachers ready to implement similar effective approaches will maximize those opportunities.

As with any intervention, assessment data are necessary to determine whether strategies are effective. Because children's response to intervention may vary across skills and measures, multiple outcome measures (as described earlier in this chapter as well as in Chapter 1) should be used. When interventions are first implemented, brief assessment indices that can be administered in a continuous fashion (e.g., curriculum-based measurement probes) are especially useful in documenting whether strategies are leading to the desired level and rate of change. In addition, a standardized norm-referenced measure, such as the Bracken Basic Concept Scale—Revised (Bracken, 1998), can be used to determine whether a child's performance is similar to that of his or her peers. These data are critical for making decisions as to continuing, discontinuing, or modifying intervention strategies. Given that many of the strategies described in this chapter have not been studied specifically for preschoolers with ADHD, it is especially important for practitioners to collect intervention outcome data when working with this population.

## PROMOTION OF ACADEMIC SKILLS CASE EXAMPLE

Aaron was a 4-year-old Caucasian boy who was referred to our early intervention program by his preschool teacher. His teacher reported that Aaron exhibited frequent problems paying attention to classroom activities, acted quickly without thinking, was subject to a high activity level, and was noncompliant with class rules and teacher commands. Aaron was the only child of a 30-year-old single mother, Ms. W., who reported similar behavior difficulties at home. A clinical interview with Ms. W. indicated that Aaron's behavior was consistent with a diagnosis of ADHD—combined type and oppositional defiant disorder (ODD). Parent and teacher ratings of Aaron's ADHD- and ODD-related behaviors were at the 98th percentile (i.e., well within the clinically significant range) for his age and gender. Aaron obtained average range scores (standard score 95% confidence interval [91, 105]) for verbal and nonverbal skills on the Differential Ability Scales. Despite average cognitive abilities, Aaron's scores on the DIBELS were low; in fact, his scores were 0 (initial sound fluency), 0 (letter naming fluency), and 1 (phoneme segmentation fluency). In a similar fashion, his Early Numeracy Skills Assessment (ENSA) quantitative concepts (total) score was 3. Not surprisingly, his Bracken Basic Concepts Scale school readiness composite score was in the below-average range (standard score of 85). Thus, Aaron was clearly in need of both behavioral and academic intervention.

In addition to Tier 3 behavioral strategies at home and school to address Aaron's ADHD- and ODD-related difficulties, several interventions were used to address his early literacy and numeracy deficits. First, as described previously (see "Strategies to Promote Early Reading Skills"), Ms. W. and Aaron's preschool teacher were encouraged to use *Ladders to Literacy* (Notari-Syverson et al., 1998) activities at home and school. Second, our consultant worked with Ms. W. to schedule shared book reading sessions for approximately 15 to 20 minutes for at least 5 nights per week. Third, Aaron's preschool teacher implemented phonemic awareness training (see Table 5.4) several times per week over 2 months. Finally, Ms. W. and Aaron's teacher employed activities at home and preschool to address Aaron's number sense skills (see "Strategies to Promote Early Mathematics Skills").

As a result of these combined strategies, Aaron exhibited considerable growth, particularly in reading skills over the subsequent 18 months. For example, his DIBELS scores in all three areas (initial sound fluency, letter naming fluency, and phoneme segmentation fluency) increased substantially over an 18-month period beginning with pretreatment (see Figure 5.3). His early numeracy skills also showed growth, albeit less dramatically, with ENSA scores increasing from 3 at pretreatment to 8 at 18 months. As a function of reading and math skill growth, Aaron's Bracken school readiness composite

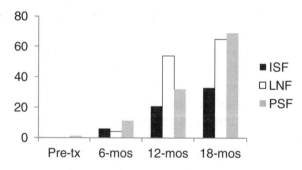

*Figure 5.3.* Scores on the Dynamic Indicators of Beginning Early Literacy Skills for Aaron as a function of treatment. ISF = initial sound fluency; LNF = letter naming fluency; PSF = phoneme segmentation fluency; tx = treatment; mos = months.

score was in the average range (standard score of 103) 18 months after beginning treatment. This readiness score was more commensurate with his cognitive ability level than what was obtained before treatment.

## CONCLUSIONS

Young children with ADHD are significantly more likely than their typically developing peers to enter elementary school with deficits in language, reading, math skills, or a combination of these. Thus, implementation of effective early intervention addressing academic skills is critical for this population. Fortunately, effective strategies for enhancing early language and reading skills have been developed for use with young children who are at risk for a variety of reasons (e.g., impoverished backgrounds). Far fewer early intervention approaches are available for addressing early math skills. In addition, there are no extant studies examining early academic intervention specifically for young children with ADHD. It will therefore be important for future research to identify effective strategies for enhancing early math skills as well as to document those academic interventions that will be most effective for young children with ADHD. In this chapter, we have assumed that those interventions found effective for other at risk groups should yield similar outcomes for children with ADHD; however, it is possible that children with this disorder may be uniquely responsive or unresponsive to specific interventions because of significant attention and hyperactivity–impulsivity difficulties. Empirical investigation of specific academic strategies with this population would shed light on this important issue.

# 6

# SAFETY AND INJURY PREVENTION

Young children with attention-deficit/hyperactivity disorder (ADHD) are at higher than average risk for accidental injuries and other medical problems (Barkley, 2006). Although a combination of variables may be responsible for this heightened risk, at least some putative underlying factors are preventable.

The purpose of this chapter is to provide an overview of the research literature demonstrating the association between early ADHD symptoms and physical injuries. We discuss possible factors underlying this association. Next, we delineate injury prevention and safety promotion strategies for use in home and preschool settings are delineated. The emphasis is on embedding prevention strategies in the ongoing parent and teacher behavioral consultation program described in previous chapters (see Chapters 3 and 4, this volume). Finally, given that research on injury prevention with the ADHD population is virtually nonexistent, we propose future directions for research and clinical practice.

# ADHD AND ACCIDENTAL INJURIES

Investigations conducted over the past several decades have demonstrated a relatively consistent association between ADHD symptomatic behaviors and risk for accidental injury (Barkley, 2006). In fact, the vast majority (57%) of children with ADHD are reported by their parents to be accident-prone, and 15% of this population have experienced four or more serious accidental injuries (Barkley, 2001). Specifically, children with ADHD are at higher than average risk for three types of injuries or medical problems: bone fractures and head injuries, burns, and accidental poisonings.

Several studies have shown that young children with ADHD, particularly boys, may be at higher risk for bone fractures, lacerations, head injuries, and other physical injuries than are control children. For example, Lee, Harrington, Chang, and Connors (2008) examined the weighted prevalence of injury (including bone fractures and head injuries) across six groups of 3- to 5-year-old children who were participants in the National Survey of Children's Health (see Blumberg et al., 2005). In addition to children identified with ADHD ($n = 191$), children in the other five groups included those with autism ($n = 82$), learning disability ($n = 307$), psychopathology ($n = 210$), other medical conditions ($n = 1802$), and nondisabled control children ($n = 13,398$). Young children with ADHD had the highest injury prevalence (26.5%) of any group, and their risk for physical injury was 2 to 3 times higher than nondisabled control children. The significantly increased risk for physical injury remained in this range even when controlling for child gender, child age, number of children living in the household, and family socioeconomic status.

Young children with ADHD may also be at risk for experiencing burn injuries requiring medical attention. Although the overall prevalence of burn injuries in this population is presumably low, some children who receive treatment in burn units appear to have exhibited significant premorbid ADHD symptoms. Thomas, Ayoub, Rosenberg, Robert, and Meyer (2004) conducted a retrospective chart review of child patients admitted to a burn care unit over a 20-year period. Of 39 children with ADHD, more than half (54%) of cases experienced a burn injury directly as a result of impulsive behavior. All but one of these young children were receiving stimulant medication before their burn injury, an indicator that their ADHD symptoms were in the moderate to high severity range.

A final medical risk for young children with ADHD is accidental ingestion of poisonous substances. For example, Szatmari, Offord, and Boyle (1989) studied the association between ADHD and various medical and psychosocial correlates in a large epidemiological sample. Two groups of children ages 4 to

16 years were compared: those with ADHD ($n$ = 157) and those without ADHD ($n$ = 2,544). A significantly higher percentage of children with ADHD (7.3%) had at least one accidental poisoning compared with those without ADHD (2.6% with at least one accidental poisoning). Interestingly, the percentage of children with ADHD who had experienced bone fractures was almost identical in the studies by Szatmari et al. (1989) and Lee et al. (2008), 23.2% and 26.5%, respectively.

Not only is there a 2 to 3 times greater risk for accidental injury associated with early childhood ADHD symptoms, but there is also evidence that injuries may be more frequent, more chronic, and more severe in this population (Barkley, 2006). Stated differently, young children with ADHD are more likely than their typically developing peers to experience injuries throughout their lifetimes, and at least some of those injuries will be relatively severe. Schwebel, Speltz, Jones, and Bardina (2002) followed 79 preschool-age boys with disruptive behavior disorders (ADHD, oppositional defiant disorder [ODD], or both) and 76 demographically matched control boys over 2 years. As found in other studies, the children with disruptive behavior disorders experienced twice the number of injuries as the matched comparison group. Further, the risk associated with ADHD symptoms extended across the 2-year period and remained even when verbal abilities and parent-rated accident proneness were taken into account. Additional studies have demonstrated that the risk for injury associated with ADHD extends to adolescence and adulthood (Jokela, Power, & Kivimäki, 2009).

The severity of injuries experienced by children with ADHD may be greater than that experienced by other children. Mangus, Bergman, Zieger, and Coleman (2004) assessed the severity of injuries experienced by children on a pediatric burn unit across a 7-year period and found that children with ADHD were significantly more likely to have had a thermal rather than flame burn, to suffer more extensive burns, and to stay for longer periods on the burn unit. Hoarea and Beattie (2003) found that children with ADHD were more likely to visit emergency rooms for their injuries (i.e., presumably because their injuries were more severe) and to experience a wider variety and greater frequency of injuries.

In fact, about one in four children with this disorder will suffer a physical injury and about one in seven an accidental poisoning at some point in their childhood. This increased injury risk remains high even when other possible contributing factors (e.g., age, gender, socioeconomic status, IQ) are taken into account. Further, children with ADHD may suffer injuries more frequently, consistently, and of greater severity than the general population.

## FACTORS ACCOUNTING FOR GREATER INJURY RISK

Several possible factors account for the greater injury risk among young children with ADHD. These factors include the presence of behaviors that constitute the core ADHD symptoms, behaviors related to comorbid disruptive behavior disorders, and lack of necessary caregiver supervision (Barkley, 2006; Lee et al., 2008). The primary reason that young children with ADHD experience injuries and/or poisonings is their higher than average rate of inattentive and hyperactive–impulsive behaviors that lead to them to take risks or not pay attention in potentially dangerous situations. Byrne, Bawden, Beattie, and DeWolfe (2003) found that the majority (58.3%) of preschoolers with ADHD displayed impulsive and inattentive behaviors that placed them at risk for physical injury. None of the control children in the Byrne et al. study displayed these behaviors to the same degree. Parents of young children with ADHD typically report that their children frequently do not pay attention while engaged in risky activities (e.g., climbing on playground equipment), ignore the possible consequences of their actions, and often choose activities that may involve risk for physical harm (Barkley, 2006). In fact, children with ADHD are 5 times more likely to engage in physically risky behaviors than their typically developing peers (Garzon, Huang, & Todd, 2008).

It is also possible that behaviors frequently associated with ADHD could increase injury risk. For example, children with this disorder frequently display difficulties with motor coordination that could lead to physical accidents (Barkley, 2006). The high rate of comorbid disruptive behavior disorders in this population could also increase risk. In fact, children with ADHD and comorbid ODD are 7 times more likely to engage in physically risky behaviors than are age-matched control children (Garzon et al., 2008). Children who are aggressive, noncompliant, and defiant are more likely to incur physical injuries than are other children (Barkley, 2006). Some researchers have speculated that aggressiveness and defiance are of greater concern than ADHD symptomatic behaviors in accounting for injury risk (e.g., Davidson, Hughes, & O'Connor, 1988). Studies also have indicated that specific injury risks may differ between children with ADHD (bone fractures) and those with ODD (burns and poisonings; Rowe, Maughan, & Goodman, 2004).

A final factor accounting for greater injury risk among young children with ADHD is inconsistent or inadequate parental monitoring of child behavior. Specifically, parents of children with this disorder may not supervise them closely when children are playing or may allow them greater freedom inside and outside the home (Davidson et al., 1988). Alternatively, when parents spend more time with their children and praise their children's appropriate behaviors more consistently, risk for physical injury may be reduced (Schwebel, Brezausek, Ramey, & Ramey, 2004). Thus, parenting behavior plays a critical role in either a negative or positive direction in determining risk for physical injuries.

All of the factors purportedly related to physical injury risk for young children with ADHD can be targeted by home- and preschool-based interventions. Specifically, treatment strategies can focus on reducing inattentive and hyperactive–impulsive behaviors; reducing or preventing aggressive, defiant actions; and promoting consistent, positive monitoring of child behavior by adults. Interventions addressing children's challenging behaviors have been described in previous chapters; however, a comprehensive early intervention protocol also should include injury prevention and safety promotion strategies.

## INJURY PREVENTION AND SAFETY PROMOTION STRATEGIES

Injury prevention and safety promotion strategies are integrated extensively throughout the early intervention for ADHD program. Specifically, promotion of child safety is targeted in one parent education session of Tier 1 intervention through the use of The Injury Prevention Program (TIPP; American Academy of Pediatrics [AAP], 1999a; http://www.aap.org/family/tippmain.htm). Parents are provided with TIPP handout materials, and behavioral consultants lead the group in discussion of safety issues and strategies. Safety-related behaviors are targeted for intervention, and parents are assigned homework (e.g., assessing risk, childproofing the home) on a regular basis following the initial injury prevention session. Safety promotion strategies are also imbedded into behavioral interventions designed as part of the preschool treatment plan. Behavioral consultants inspect homes and preschools for safety risks and childproofing when conducting home visits and school consultations. Finally, use of safety promotion strategies is assessed on a regular basis through parent surveys and behavioral consultant observation.

### Parent Education

The entire seventh session of Tier 1 parent education (see Chapter 3) is devoted to safety promotion and injury prevention. The objectives of this session are to (a) increase parental awareness of potential safety hazards in the home and neighborhood, (b) enhance understanding of prevention strategies and emergency procedures, (c) encourage self-assessment of safety hazards currently present in the home, and (d) increase use of injury prevention and safety promotion strategies in the home. Three primary topic areas are covered: the importance of injury prevention for young children with ADHD, potential safety hazards and specific prevention strategies, and general prevention strategies. Parents are provided numerous handouts regarding safety promotion activities from the TIPP, as well as information from the American Red Cross and local poison control center about procedures to use in case of emergency. They are also given a list of materials that should be kept in a first-aid kit (e.g., bandage tape, tweezers, cold pack, sealed container of antiseptic). Behavioral consultants consistently emphasize the use of proactive strategies that require parents to anticipate potential hazards and alter the environment to reduce risk before children have an opportunity for injury.

The first step in parent education is to inform parents of the higher risk for injury associated with ADHD. Research documenting this increased risk, as discussed previously in this chapter, is presented in clear, frank terms to ensure parental understanding. In particular, it is emphasized that injury risk is heightened not only because of children's inattentive and hyperactive–impulsive behaviors but also because of lack of awareness and supervision by parents and other adult caretakers. Parents are reminded that children's behaviors are targeted by intervention strategies designed through parent education and behavioral consultation; however, it is equally important that parents increase their awareness of possible hazardous situations and more consistently supervise their children's behaviors. Most injuries are predictable and are, therefore, preventable. Measures to prevent injuries are relatively easy to employ and are critically important for parents of young children with ADHD.

The majority of this parent education session is devoted to delineating specific hazardous situations and objects followed by discussing specific actions that parents can take to prevent injuries in these situations (see Table 6.1). The most common and concerning safety risks for young children with ADHD include falls, poison ingestion, fire and burn hazards, toy-related injuries, choking on food or other objects, car injuries, bicycle accidents, pedestrian accidents, water accidents, and gun accidents. Specific safety promotion strategies are adapted from the TIPP program available from the AAP.

Young children can experience falls in a number of settings but most prominently when playing in the home or outdoors, as well as when riding a bicycle, tricycle, scooter, or skateboard. Parents are encouraged to use several strategies to prevent falls (see Exhibit 6.1). In the home setting, furniture should be arranged away from potential hazards, such as windows or loose cabinets and bookcases. Children should not be allowed to play around balconies, fire escapes, or stair landings. Safety gates can be used to enclose play areas or to cordon off areas that could cause injuries in a fall (e.g., brick fireplace). Children should be closely supervised around stairs or when playing in elevated areas (e.g., playground equipment). Proper attire should be worn while playing so that children are less likely to trip and fall. Further, parents should set boundaries for safe play zones and then closely supervise children so that these boundaries are maintained.

TABLE 6.1
Most Common Safety Risks and Associated Prevention Strategies

| Safety risk | Possible prevention strategies |
| --- | --- |
| Falls | Arrange furniture away from dangerous objects |
| | Install window guards |
| | Safeguard play areas |
| Poison ingestion | Safe storage |
| | Teach children precautions |
| | Follow label recommendations |
| | Have poison aid agents available |
| Fire and burn hazards | Close supervision around fires and other burn hazards (e.g., stove) |
| | Install smoke detectors |
| | Plan and teach escape routes |
| | Monitor water temperature |
| | Keep fire-starting materials locked and out of reach and sight |
| | Use electrical socket covers |
| Toy-related injuries | Select age-appropriate and safe toys |
| | Monitor condition of toys |
| | Pay attention to safety recommendation labels |
| Choking | Arrange structured times for eating and snacking |
| | Make sure child is sitting down while eating |
| | Recognize choking symptoms |
| | Use Heimlich maneuver when necessary |
| Car injuries | Properly install and consistently use age-appropriate car safety seat |
| | Children should ride in back seat |
| | Attach both harness and seat belt securely |
| Bicycle accidents | Always use helmet |
| | Teach "rules of the road" |
| | Make sure bicycle is of appropriate size and is well maintained |
| Pedestrian accidents | Teach pedestrian safety skills |
| | Teach children to use caution when crossing streets |
| | Supervise sidewalk and street behavior |
| Water accidents | Never leave unattended, no matter how shallow |
| | Pay attention to open water |
| | Provide access to swimming lessons |
| | Enforce water safety rules |
| | Learn child cardiopulmonary resuscitation (CPR) |
| Gun accidents | Unload and lock guns |
| | Store ammunition in a place different from gun |
| | Use trigger locks |

Children age 5 and under are at greatest risk for nonfatal poisoning and account for the majority of all poisoning exposures. Thus, parents are asked to conduct a home inventory of potential risk for accidental poisoning using the poison lookout checklist in Appendix 6.1. Potentially poisonous substances that could be accidentally ingested include personal care products, lead paint,

EXHIBIT 6.1
Fall Prevention Strategies

1. Use playground equipment that is safe and well maintained. The surface under and around equipment should be soft and shock-absorbent.
2. Use durable, balanced furniture that will not tip over easily.
3. Place safety gates at top and bottom of stairs.
4. Install window guards on upstairs windows.
5. Pick up toys and other objects from the floor and clean up spills quickly.
6. Secure and remove loose mats and rugs.
7. Use skid-proof mats or stickers in bathtub area.
8. Keep play areas well lit.
9. Do not allow children to climb on furniture, stools, or ladders. Discourage indoor running.
10. Teach children how to play safely, involve them in making rules for playground behavior, monitor their behavior, and enforce rules consistently.

From *Health and Safety in the Child Care Setting: Prevention of Injuries* (p. 56–57), by the California Child Care Health Program, 1998. Berkeley, CA: Author. Copyright 1998 by the California Child Care Health Program. Adapted with permission.

medicines or vitamins, and plants. The most important preventive strategy is to store all household items, medications, and other toxic products out of children's reach and sight, preferably in a locked cabinet. Parents should teach children to take precautions with toxic substances; stickers that clearly demarcate poisons (e.g., skull and crossbones or Mr. Yuk symbol) can aid in this process (see Appendix 6.2). Parents should make sure that medications and other toxic substances are stored in containers that have safety caps and should follow label recommendations when using these substances. Replacing lead-based paint in the home can reduce the potential for lead exposure. Ipecac and other poison aid agents should be kept in the home in the event that children ingest a toxic substance (see Appendix 6.2). Parents should be cautioned to use poison aid agents only on the advice of a physician or poison control agent. Emergency telephone numbers (including poison control) should be kept handy, and children should be taught to use these numbers as soon as they can understand that process.

Young children are particularly vulnerable to fires and burn injuries because of their curiosity and ignorance of potential dangers. Children with ADHD are at even higher risk because they may not attend to fire and burn hazards in their environment or may engage in risky, impulsive behavior around such hazards. As is the case for toxic substances, all fire-starting materials (e.g., matches, lighters) should be kept out of children's reach and sight, preferably in a locked container. Electrical socket covers should be used throughout the home. Water heater temperature should be set at a safe level to prevent accidental scalding during baths or showers. Smoke detectors should be installed on all levels of the home, and children should be taught to react appropriately to detector signals by using escape routes from the home. Children should not be allowed near stoves or other cooking areas unless they are closely supervised. Finally, homes should be safety proofed by eliminating any dangling cords and exposed, frayed electrical wires.

Common toy-related injuries include choking and falling. Fortunately, most of these injuries are relatively minor and can be prevented. Parents are provided with a toy safety checklist that lists important considerations when choosing and evaluating toys for safety (see Appendix 6.3). The most important prevention strategy is to choose toys carefully by following age and safety recommendation labels. In addition, toys should be kept in good condition, and those that have broken parts that could be dangerous should be discarded and replaced. Finally, parents are encouraged to play with their children, especially when they are using a toy for the first time. This allows parents to observe whether any safety hazards may be present and monitor children's behavior to minimize injury.

Choking can occur not only with toys but also with other small objects and food (e.g., grapes, hot dogs, peanuts). Sometimes choking can occur because children are moving while eating or are putting large amounts of food in their mouths. To some extent, having children eat and snack under more structured conditions (e.g., eating at a set time and place) can prevent activity-related choking incidents. Specifically, parents need to ensure that children are sitting while eating and monitor the amounts of food that they put in their mouths, if the latter is an issue. The symptoms of choking are reviewed with parents so that they can act quickly with first aid, if necessary. Signs of choking include difficulty breathing or speaking, inability to cough, wheezing, clutching of throat or gesturing, bluish facial complexion, confusion, and unexplained loss of consciousness. Parents are provided with a handout from the American Red Cross that reviews first aid for choking situations (e.g., encouraging the child to keep coughing, using the Heimlich maneuver if the child cannot breathe or speak). Parents are also encouraged to take a CPR course through their local Red Cross chapter.

Young children with ADHD can be at risk for car-related injuries not only because of vehicular accidents but also because of excessive movement in the car (e.g., falling from the seat or colliding with the door or window). Parents are provided with a handout that includes 10 tips for car safety (from http://www.seatcheck.org) that emphasizes using properly installed car seats that are always placed in the back seat. Parents are asked to bring their children's car seats to this training session so that consultants can ensure that families are using the proper seats based on children's age and weight. Further, the proper use of these seats is reviewed (e.g., always attach both the shoulder harness and seat belt securely to the car seat).

The risk of sustaining injury is increased when children begin riding bicycles, scooters, and skateboards. It is critical for parents to ensure that children wear helmets any time they are riding a bicycle, even as a passenger in a seat on an adult's bicycle. Getting children to comply with this rule may be easier when parents model this behavior by also wearing helmets when riding. Children should be dressed in attire that does not interfere with the operation of the bicycle. Further, the bicycle should be an appropriate size for the child's height and age. As is the case with toys, it is important that bicycles are in good condition and are not hazardous to ride. When children are first learning to ride a bicycle, parents should teach, prompt, and reinforce following the "rules of the road" (e.g., using proper hand signals). Finally, it is important for parents to supervise children while they are riding and to ensure that they are only riding in safe (i.e., relatively traffic-free) environments.

Children may also sustain injuries as pedestrians when crossing streets or walking or running on a sidewalk. Thus, parents are strongly encouraged to supervise all play that occurs near streets and driveways. Further, parents should teach, prompt, and reinforce following pedestrian rules (e.g., wait for adult to cross the street, look both ways before crossing). If children eventually walk to and from elementary school, these rules become even more critical to monitor.

Water safety is another important area in an injury prevention program. Unfortunately, young children can drown in as little as an inch or two of water in a very short period of time. Swimming pools are potentially hazardous, but so are wading pools, bathtubs, hot tubs, toilets, and even buckets. Thus, the importance of never leaving children unattended near water, no matter how shallow, must be emphasized with parents. In addition, all water containers should be kept out of reach, and toilet lids should be shut and locked, if possible. Children should be taught to have a healthy respect for water and should receive swimming lessons as early in life as possible. Water safety rules (e.g., always swim in pairs, swim within sight of an adult) must be taught, prompted, and reinforced on a regular basis. Finally, parents should be aware of emergency procedures and learn CPR, if possible.

A final injury risk is present in homes where firearms are kept. Basic gun safety rules should be reviewed with parents. First, parents must realize that no guns are safe for young children to handle, even when an adult is supervising. Second, all firearms should be locked in a safe, secure place and kept unloaded. Ammunition should be stored separately, preferably in a locked container. Finally, trigger locks should be installed on all firearms.

The final component of the parent education session focused on safety promotion involves discussion of a general prevention plan adapted from the TIPP (AAP, 1999a). The plan comprises four overarching strategies. First, parents should supervise children's behavior at all times, especially when they are playing in potentially dangerous settings. Children should never be left alone in such situations, even for a minute or two. Second, as much as possible, potential hazards should be removed from the home or secured in locked, out-of-reach locations. Third, parents should always plan ahead when entering a setting that might be hazardous (e.g., swimming pool) or before children engaging in potentially dangerous activities (e.g., riding a bicycle, playing on playground equipment). In addition to paying close attention to children's behavior, parents should also have a plan for handling any emergency that may arise. Finally, children should be taught safety rules by establishing clear, firm, and consistent guidelines for activities that might be physically risky. Rule-following behavior in these situations should serve as targets for behavioral interventions so that consistent consequences are available for following or breaking rules.

Parents are also provided with several advisories regarding child care and babysitting. For example, although older siblings may be responsible babysitters for typically developing children, siblings are not usually good choices to take care of young children with ADHD because of the potential risks involved with this population. Thus, experienced caregivers, especially those who have babysat for other children with ADHD, are preferred. Finally, it is critical that parents know where their children are at all times and periodically check in with babysitters to ensure this knowledge.

## Behavioral Intervention Strategies

Although a training session can arm parents with information about effective injury prevention strategies, information alone is rarely sufficient to change behavior (Kazdin, 2001). Thus, consultants review safety promotion methods periodically (e.g., in alternate training sessions) throughout the parent education program. Further, if Tier 3 intervention is necessary, then injury-related behaviors can serve as targets for assessment-based intervention developed through behavioral consultation as described in chapter 3. For example, "safe play behavior" (e.g., following parent safety rules and cooperating with other children) can be taught, prompted, and reinforced in home and playground settings. In this fashion, injury prevention strategies can be individualized based on the specific risks present in a given home setting, based on the behavioral risks exhibited by individual children, or both. Consultants can then support and reinforce parent implementation of safety and injury prevention guidelines taught during parent education sessions as part of the behavior support plan.

## Extension to Preschool Classroom

Clearly, many of the same injury risks encountered at home are also present in the preschool. In fact, injury risk may be greater given the number of children present and the potential hazards encountered particularly during free play activities. Thus, safety promotion and injury prevention strategies should also be used in preschool classroom and playground settings. As was the case for the home setting, a two-pronged approach should be used. First, teachers are provided with information to alert them to potential injury hazards in the classroom and on the playground. Primary risks include falls during play activities, toy-related injuries, choking while eating, pedestrian accidents, and possibly poison ingestion. Similar prevention strategies to those provided as part of parent education are recommended to address these risks. Second, safety promotion strategies are individualized on the basis of potential hazards observed in the specific preschool as well as the specific risky behaviors exhibited by children. As such, specific child behaviors can be incorporated into the behavior management plan implemented by preschool teachers in the context of assessment-based intervention (i.e., Tier 3 as discussed in Chapter 4). Consultants work with teachers to teach children safety rules, prompt safe behavior during play and other activities, and reinforce adherence with safety rules. It is particularly ideal if the same safety-related behaviors can be targeted in both home and preschool environments, thus promoting consistency and support across settings. The use of consistent strategies across settings and caretakers presumably increases the chances that safe behavior will be generalized across environments (even when caretakers are not present) and maintained over time.

### Periodic Assessment and Modification

Several assessment strategies are used to document potential hazards in the home environment and the degree to which parents have been successful in adopting injury prevention recommendations. At the beginning of the seventh parent education session (i.e., when safety promotion and injury prevention are discussed), parents complete the TIPP Safety Survey: From 1 to 4 Years (Parts 1 and 2; AAP, 1999b). This 50-item survey asks parents to report the relative safety of the current home environment as well as the degree to which injury prevention methods are used. Sample items include the following: "Do you keep electrical appliances and cords out of child's reach?"; "Does child play in the driveway or street?" "Does child wear a helmet when riding a bike?" Survey results serve as baseline data to gauge the degree of change following parent education and behavioral consultation. This survey is completed periodically (e.g., every 6 months), and behavioral consultants review results with parents as a vehicle to reinforce appropriately implemented strategies and prompt use of prevention techniques not currently in place. Parents are encouraged to consult handout materials and conduct more frequent self-assessments using the TIPP Safety Survey as a way to promote continuous use of injury prevention methods.

As described in Chapter 3, if Tier 3 intervention is warranted, behavioral consultants make periodic home visits to facilitate development and implementation of assessment-based intervention. During these visits, consultants informally assess whether potential safety hazards exist and recommend changes address injury risks. Also, consultants complete the Early Childhood Home Observation for Measurement of the Environment (EC-HOME; Caldwell & Bradley, 2001) every 3 to 6 months. The EC-HOME contains eight subscales (e.g., learning materials, language stimulation, academic stimulation) that assess the degree to which home settings are conducive to age-appropriate child development and learning. One of the subscales (i.e., Physical Environment) includes items related to safety (e.g., building appears safe and free of hazards), and these can serve as another check on the degree to which injury prevention methods are used by parents. Finally, to the extent that child and parent behaviors related to injury prevention (e.g., child compliance with household safety rules) are targeted through assessment-based intervention, changes in these behaviors are assessed on a continuous basis, similar to other intervention targets.

Consultants use these assessment data to reinforce parental efforts at injury prevention and to suggest modifications, as necessary. Specifically, parents are encouraged to use procedures that are not currently in place and are given suggestions for changes to strategies that are not being used appropriately or are only partially implemented. Further, with maturation, children's interests and activities will change, thus requiring ongoing appraisal of new potential injury risks. For example, as children are able to begin riding a bicycle or skateboard, safety promotion procedures related to these activities become critical to implement. Thus, parents are reminded of changes in risk that are associated with children's ongoing development. The overarching goal is for parents to think proactively about safety and anticipate potential hazards and risks before they occur.

### Safety and Injury Prevention Case Example

David was a 3-year-old African American boy who was referred to our early intervention program by his pediatrician because of concerns about his highly impulsive and active behavior. David lived with his parents, Mr. and Mrs. Z., as well as his older brother and younger sister. He attended a preschool program three mornings per week. According to parent and teacher ratings as well as clinical interview data, David's challenging behaviors were consistent with ADHD—combined type and ODD. On a positive note, his cognitive abilities were in the high average range (Standard Score of 112 on the Differential Ability Scales), and he was making developmentally appropriate progress in terms of early literacy and numeracy skills.

Mr. and Mrs. Z. reported David to be highly "accident prone," presumably because of his high activity level and proclivity to act quickly without considering consequences. In fact, they described him as a daredevil who was fearless on the playground. As a result, they had made several emergency room visits with him over the previous 18 months for a broken hand and for two separate injuries that required stitches on his head and foot. The consultant working with Mr. and Mrs. Z. conducted a safety survey of their home and also reviewed the typical setting and antecedent events surrounding David's injuries. This assessment indicated that (a) Mr. and Mrs. Z. rarely reminded David of safety rules before he played outside and only intermittently supervised his play behavior, (b) Mr. and Mrs. Z. frequently allowed David to climb on play equipment that was not developmentally appropriate (e.g., tall jungle gym), and (c) David incurred most injuries while attempting to show off his daring behavior to impress other children on the playground.

On the basis of this assessment, the consultant and David's parents developed a safety promotion plan that involved several components. First, David was allowed to play outdoors with other children only when an adult was available to supervise his behavior closely. Second, he was allowed to play only on equipment that was deemed developmentally appropriate and safe. They did not take him to playgrounds that included larger equipment that was potentially dangerous. Third, Mr. and Mrs. Z. reviewed safety rules with David before each outdoor play session. If David was observed to follow these rules on a consistent basis, he was then provided with positive reinforcement (i.e., parental praise and access to a preferred toy for a specified period of time). Finally, the consultant worked with Mr. and Mrs. Z. to teach David behaviors that he could employ to make friends and gain peer attention when playing with groups of children. These social initiation behaviors presumably could serve the same function as his daring attempts to gain peer attention.

As part of our early intervention program, Mr. and Mrs. Z. completed the TIPP Safety Survey every 6 months beginning with a pretreatment assessment. Before implementation of the safety promotion plan, David's TIPP score was relatively low (i.e., score of 98 compared with a mean score of 119.3 for our early intervention sample). After several months of Mr. and Mrs. Z. using the safety promotion plan, David's scores increased and were slightly above the mean for the ADHD sample as a whole (see Figure 6.1). These high scores were maintained at the 12- and 18-month assessments.

## CONCLUSIONS AND FUTURE DIRECTIONS

Young children with ADHD are at higher than average risk for accidental injuries and poisonings because of their impulsive, risky behavior and comorbid behavior difficulties, as well as the lack of consistent parental supervision. Thus,

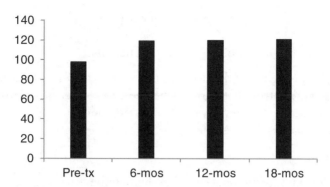

*Figure 6.1.* Total score on The Injury Prevention Plan (TIPP) safety survey for David as a function of treatment. Note that higher scores indicate better injury prevention. tx = treatment; mos = months.

comprehensive early intervention should address these risks by implementing prevention strategies in home and preschool settings. Our early intervention program involves a two-pronged approach in both settings: (a) education regarding the most common injury hazards and requisite prevention activities and (b) consultation regarding assessment-based intervention to target the most prominent risky behaviors engaged in or situations encountered by individual children. Safety promotion and injury prevention strategies are modified over time on the basis of child developmental changes as well as assessment data reflecting the degree to which strategies have been successful. As with other aspects (e.g., assessment-based intervention) of our early intervention program, it is important that strategies and procedures are consistent across care providers and settings. The use of a consistent approach may lead to greater generalization and maintenance of safety-promoting behaviors.

Although the risk for injury associated with ADHD in home settings has been well documented, few, if any, studies have specifically examined ADHD-related injury risk in preschool classrooms and playgrounds. The risks in homes and preschools are presumably similar; however, it would be helpful to have more specific documentation of how risks may differ across settings and whether there are additional hazards present in preschool environments not encountered in the home setting.

Research studies are also needed to document the degree to which specific prevention strategies are effective in reducing risk for specific injuries. Our two-pronged approach to safety promotion is part of a larger, comprehensive early intervention protocol. Thus, our outcome data do not allow us to parcel out which strategy or combination of strategies was the "active ingredient" in reducing injury risk. More specific intervention outcome studies could lead to a more parsimonious, cost-effective approach to injury prevention. Feasibility and cost-efficiency could enhance acceptability and implementation by practitioners.

# APPENDIX 6.1

## Poison Lookout Checklist

The home areas listed below are the most common sites of accidental poisonings. Follow this checklist to learn how to correct situations that may lead to poisonings. If you answer "No" to any questions, fix the situation quickly. Your goal is to have all of your answers "Yes."

**The Kitchen**                                                      Yes        No

1. Do all harmful products in the cabinets have        _____      _____
   child-resistant caps? Products like furniture pol-
   ish, drain cleaners and some oven cleaners should
   have safety packaging to keep little children from
   accidentally opening the packages.
2. Are all potentially harmful products in their       _____      _____
   original containers? There are two dangers if
   products aren't stored in their original containers. Labels on the original containers often give
   first aid information if someone should swallow
   the product. And, if products are stored in containers like drinking glasses or soda bottles,
   someone may think it is food and swallow the
   poison.
3. Are the harmful products stored away from food?     _____      _____
   If harmful products are placed next to food,
   someone may accidentally get food and a poison
   mixed up and swallow the poison.
4. Have all potentially harmful products been put      _____      _____
   up high and out of reach of children? The best
   way to prevent poisoning is making sure that it's
   impossible to find and get at the poisons. Locking
   all cabinets that hold dangerous products is the
   best poison prevention.

**The Bathroom**
1. Did you ever stop to think that medicines could     _____      _____
   be poison if used improperly? Many children are
   poisoned each year by overdoses of aspirin. If
   aspirin can poison, just think of how many other
   poisons might be in your medicine cabinet.

**The Bathroom** (*Continued*)                                    Yes        No

2. Do your aspirins and other potentially harmful products have child-resistant closures? Aspirins and most prescription drugs come with child-resistant caps. Check to see if yours have them, and that they are properly secured. Check your prescriptions before leaving the pharmacy to make sure the medicines are in child-resistant packaging.                           \_\_\_\_\_      \_\_\_\_\_

3. Have you thrown out all out-of-date prescriptions? As medicines get older, the chemicals inside of them can change. So what was once a good medicine may now be a dangerous poison. Flush all old drugs down the toilet. Rinse the container well, and then discard it.            \_\_\_\_\_      \_\_\_\_\_

4. Are all medicines in their original containers with original labels? Prescription medicines may or may not list ingredients. The prescription number on the label will, however, allow rapid identification of the ingredients by the pharmacist should they not be listed.             \_\_\_\_\_      \_\_\_\_\_

5. If your vitamins or vitamin/mineral supplements contain iron, are they in child-resistant packaging? Most people think of vitamins and minerals as foods and, therefore nontoxic, but a few iron pills can seriously harm a child.            \_\_\_\_\_      \_\_\_\_\_

**The Garage or Storage Area**

1. Did you know that many things in your garage or storage area that can be swallowed are terrible poisons? Death can occur when people swallow everyday substances such as charcoal lighter, paint thinner and remover, and antifreeze and turpentine.           \_\_\_\_\_      \_\_\_\_\_

2. Do all these poisons in your garage/storage area have child-resistant caps?           \_\_\_\_\_      \_\_\_\_\_

3. Are they stored in the original containers?           \_\_\_\_\_      \_\_\_\_\_

4. Are the original labels on the containers?           \_\_\_\_\_      \_\_\_\_\_

**The Garage or Storage Area** (*Continued*)                    Yes          No

  5. Have you made sure that no poisons are stored          ____        ____
     in drinking glasses or soda bottles?
  6. Are all of these harmful products locked up and        ____        ____
     out of sight and reach from your children?

**When all of your answers are "YES," then continue this level of poison protection by making sure whenever you buy potentially harmful products that they have child-resistant closures and are kept out of sight and reach.**

*Note.* From U.S. Consumer Product Safety Commission Publication No. 383. In the public domain.

## APPENDIX 6.2: FOR POISON CONTROL, USE MR. YUK

Mr. Yuk is the poison warning symbol used by many poison centers throughout the United States.

Mr. Yuk stickers say "No!" to little children who can't read warning labels on many dangerous products in your home.

Children are naturally curious. They touch, smell, and taste things as a natural part of learning. Your home is filled with many products that make life easier and more pleasant, such as cleaning supplies, cosmetics, and medications. Any of these products can poison a child who ingests or inhales it.

Teach your child that Mr. Yuk means *NO!* Allow children to watch as you place Mr. Yuk stickers on dangerous products. Place a Mr. Yuk sticker on your telephone—the name and telephone number of your nearest poison center surround Mr. Yuk's face.

And remember, if you suspect a poisoning, call your poison center immediately. Expert medical staff are there 24 hours a day, 7 days a week to give you prompt, reliable help.

**There should be a bottle of syrup of Ipecac in every home.**

**Syrup of Ipecac is a medicine for emergency use in poisoning. When given to a child or an adult, it causes vomiting. Syrup of Ipecac can be purchased in any drug store. It does not need a prescription.**

**Never give syrup of Ipecac without calling your poison center first.**

**Poison center staff will give you clear directions for its use if it is necessary.**

**Put Mr. Yuk on products like these:**

| | |
|---|---|
| Acids | Copper and brass |
| Aerosols | Corn and wart remover |
| Ammonia | Dandruff shampoo |
| Antifreeze | Dishwasher detergent |
| Antiseptics | Drain cleaners |
| Aspirin | Drugs |
| Baby oil | Epoxy glue |
| Bathroom bowl cleaner | Eye makeup |
| Bleach | Furniture polish |
| Benzene | Garden sprays |
| Bubble bath | Gun cleaners |
| Carbon tetrachloride | Hair dryers |
| Cigarettes | Herbicides |
| Cleaner | Insecticides |
| Cleaning fluids | Iodine |
| Cologne | Kerosene |

Mace (chemical)
Model cement
Nail polish remover
Narcotics
Oven cleaner
Paint/paint thinner
Pesticides
Pine oil

Rodenticides
Rubbing alcohol
Shaving lotion
Silver polish
Strychnine
Turpentine
Vitamins
Window wash solvent

## APPENDIX 6.3: TOYS: SAFETY CHECKLIST FOR PRESCHOOLERS

The following guidelines should be used when considering toys for preschool-age children.

- The toy is not too heavy for your child's strength.
- The toy is well constructed. (A poorly made toy can break or come apart, easily exposing hazards such as wires or springs.)
- The toy does not have sharp edges that can cut or scratch.
- All parts of the toy, including print and decoration, are nonpoisonous.
- Old baby furniture and toys have not been painted or repainted with lead-base paint.
- There are no slots or holes that can pinch your child's fingers.
- No part of the toy, such as a doll's hair bow, is attached with a straight pin or staple.
- All moving parts are securely attached.
- A broken toy is repaired or thrown away.
- Indoor toys remain indoors so they do not rust.
- The windup mechanism in a mechanical toy is enclosed to avoid catching hair, fingers, and clothing.
- All riding toys are well constructed and well balanced.
- The wheels on riding toys are large, sturdy, and spaced far apart.
- A stuffed doll or animal is made with strong material and thread and not filled with small, loose pellets.
- Toys made with cloth carry the labels *flame resistant*, *flame retardant*, or *nonflammable*.

# 7

# PSYCHOTROPIC MEDICATION TREATMENT

One of the most common treatments for attention-deficit/hyperactivity disorder (ADHD) in the school-age population is psychotropic medication. Several compounds are used, including various central nervous system (CNS) stimulants as well as a few nonstimulant medications (see Table 7.1). Given the success of these medications in treating symptoms of ADHD in school-age children, since the 1990s there has been a precipitous increase in pharmacotherapy for treating this disorder in young children (Rappley, 2006). In fact, the use of stimulants for preschool children enrolled in state Medicaid programs doubled over the 6-year period 1992–1998 (Rushton & Whitmire, 2001). Further, approximately 67% of day care centers in one state reported giving medication to young children for ADHD (Sinkovits, Kelly, & Ernst, 2003).

The growing use of psychotropic medication to treat ADHD symptoms in young children is not surprising given the established efficacy of pharmacotherapy for older children and adolescents with this disorder (for a review, see Barkley, 2006). CNS stimulants, such as methylphenidate (MPH), have been studied since the 1960s and have been consistently associated with improvements in attention and impulse control for the majority of children treated (Connor, 2006a). More recently, nonstimulant compounds such as atomoxetine, clonidine, and guanfacine have also been found to reduce

TABLE 7.1
Medications Used to Treat Attention-Deficit/Hyperactivity Disorder

| Class of medication | Medication compound |
|---|---|
| Central nervous system stimulants | methylphenidate—short acting or immediate release (e.g., Ritalin, Focalin, Methylin) methylphenidate—long acting or extended release (e.g., Concerta, Focalin XR, Ritalin LA, Metadate CD) dextroamphetamine (Dexedrine) mixed amphetamine (Adderall) lisdexamfetamine (Vyvanse) |
| Nonstimulants | atomoxetine (Strattera) clonidine (Catapres) guanfacine (Intuniv) |

ADHD symptoms; however, the effects of these drugs appear to be weaker than those found for stimulants (Connor, 2006b; Spencer, 2006). In some cases, these medications also enhance academic and social functioning, although these effects are not consistently found across studies, nor are outcomes "normalized" relative to the general population (Brown et al., 2007).

The purpose of this chapter is to provide an overview of medication treatment for ADHD in young children. First, we review medication studies conducted with this age group, with particular emphasis on symptomatic outcome, impact on functioning, and possible adverse side effects. Next, we describe methods for determining whether medication is necessary in treating young children with ADHD. Third, we delineate procedures and measures for assessing medication effects to help physicians and families decide whether pharmacotherapy is helpful and which dosage of medication is optimal. Finally, we offer recommendations regarding the appropriate use of medication in young children as well as important directions for future research in this area. Although psychotropic medication, especially CNS stimulants, is considered a first-line treatment for ADHD in older children and adolescents, pharmacotherapy is a secondary option for treatment of this disorder in young children. Stated differently, psychosocial (primarily behavioral) interventions are the primary treatment choice to address ADHD symptoms in preschool-age children.

EFFECTS OF MEDICATION ON YOUNG CHILDREN WITH ADHD

A variety of psychotropic medications have been investigated as possible treatment for ADHD symptoms in young children. Compounds have included MPH and other CNS stimulants, atomoxetine, fluoxetine, clonidine, and guanfacine. Ghuman, Arnold, and Anthony (2008) conducted a systematic review of the medication literature relevant to young children with ADHD and located 24 published studies during the period 1967–2007, the vast majority of which were investigations of CNS stimulants. In fact, there are no controlled studies of nonstimulant medications in this age group, and thus the efficacy of nonstimulants for treating preschoolers with ADHD is essentially unknown. Although findings have differed across individual studies, most placebo-controlled investigations of stimulants have shown significant reductions in ratings and observations of ADHD-related behaviors, with approximately 80% of treated children showing a positive response (Ghuman et al., 2008). Until recently, however, most studies used relatively small samples and limited outcome measures.

The most comprehensive study of stimulant medication (MPH) for young children with ADHD is the Preschool ADHD Treatment Study (PATS; Kollins et al., 2006). A sample of 303 children (76% boys) between 3.0 and 5.5 years old who met *Diagnostic and Statistical Manual of Mental Disorders* (4th ed., text revision; American Psychiatric Association, 2000) criteria for ADHD were initially enrolled in the study. It is important to note that participating children went through several phases before the controlled medication trial phase, including screening, parent education, and open-label safety lead-in. These three phases were included to (a) ensure that children met comprehensive inclusion criteria establishing an ADHD diagnosis; (b) gauge children's response to psychosocial treatment (i.e., parent training) with positive responders not participating in medication trials; and (c) verify that children would tolerate MPH, and those children showing moderate to severe adverse side effects with a relatively low dosage (below 5 milligrams) did not continue in the study. For example, of the 261 children whose families completed the 10-week parent training (using the Community Parent Education program; C. E. Cunningham, Bremner, & Secord, 1998), 37 (14%) exhibited sufficient improvement such that parents no longer sought medication treatment (Greenhill et al., 2006). An additional 45 (17%) children withdrew following parent training because parents did not want medication, children no longer met inclusion criteria, or families moved and were lost to follow-up. Sixteen children withdrew during or following the open-label safety lead-in phase, leaving 165 children who were enrolled in the placebo-controlled crossover medication trial (147 of whom completed the trial).

A comprehensive set of parent and teacher rating scales along with direct observations of classroom behavior were used to examine the overall efficacy of MPH and specific dose–response effects (Kollins et al., 2006). Children who participated in the 9-week controlled medication trial phase were assessed across 5 weeks of dosage titration (placebo, 1.25 milligrams, 2.5 milligrams, 5 milligrams, and 7.5 milligrams) with each dosage used for 1 week. An optimal dosage was determined for each child, who then completed a 4-week controlled parallel study phase in which children were randomly assigned to receive either placebo or their optimal MPH dosage. During the 5-week crossover phase (in which each child received a different MPH dosage or placebo each week), statistically significant reductions in combined parent and teacher ratings of ADHD symptoms relative to placebo were found for the three highest dosages (i.e., all dosages except 1.25 milligrams; Greenhill et al., 2006). Symptoms ratings did not differ among the three highest dosages; however, there was a significant linear dose–response effect indicating step-wise reductions in ADHD symptoms as dosage increased. The magnitude of symptom reduction effects relative to placebo was in the small to moderate range (effect size ranged from 0.16 to 0.72), which contrasts with moderate to large effects for MPH found for elementary school–age children with ADHD (e.g., MTA Cooperative Group, 1999). However, Ghuman et al. (2007) found moderate to large effect sizes favoring MPH over placebo for children with no or one comorbid disorder (most frequently oppositional defiant disorder [ODD]). Children with ADHD and two or more comorbid disorders showed smaller magnitude of MPH effects.

As has been found for older children with ADHD treated with stimulants (e.g., Rapport, Denney, DuPaul, & Gardner, 1994), these group-level findings for MPH effects are qualified by substantial differences in medication response across individuals. Specifically, relatively equal percentages of children (ranging between 15% and 22%) were found to show optimal responses to each of the four active MPH dosages. Further, 12% of the children were found to show either no response or optimal response to placebo rather than an active dose of MPH. The latter children did not continue participating in the 4-week parallel study phase, along with an additional 26 children who showed behavior deterioration, significant adverse side effects, declined further participation, or were lost to follow-up.

A sample of 114 children entered the 4-week parallel medication phase, of whom 77 completed all 4 weeks (Greenhill et al., 2006). Not surprisingly, children who received their optimal MPH dosage obtained significantly lower parent and teacher ADHD symptom ratings than did children who received placebo. The effect sizes for each dosage (relative to placebo) were once again in the low to moderate range. These efficacy outcomes are tempered by the fact that there was substantial attrition during this phase, primarily due to lack of medication response. Further, only 22% of children assigned to their optimal dosage were found to exhibit investigator-defined criteria for "excellent" response compared with 13% of children receiving placebo. This difference in percentage of excellent responders was not statistically significant.

Side effects were systematically assessed during all medication phases of the PATS, primarily through clinician ratings based on parent and teacher reports. Approximately 30% of parents reported that their children exhibited moderate to severe adverse side effects during one or more of the active medication phases (Wigal et al., 2006). As has been found for older children with ADHD (see Connor, 2006a), the three most commonly reported adverse side effects included decreased appetite, trouble sleeping, and weight loss. All three of these side effects occurred significantly more often during MPH than placebo conditions. Twenty-one children (11%) discontinued participation in the study because of medication-induced adverse side effects. Of additional concern, for the 95 children who remained on MPH following the controlled medication phases of the study, annual growth rates were 20% below expectations for height and 55.2% less than expected for weight (Swanson et al., 2006). Thus, the use of stimulant medication in this age group must be considered by balancing possible benefits of symptom reduction against probable reductions in growth velocity, although long-term studies of growth reduction are scarce.

Few studies have examined the impact of MPH and other stimulants on the early academic skills and social functioning of preschoolers with ADHD. Children who received their optimal MPH dosage during the 4-week parallel medication phase of the PATS were rated as more socially competent by their teachers and as showing global improvement by their clinicians relative to children who received placebo (Abikoff et al., 2007). Effect sizes were in the moderate range for these group differences. Alternatively, medication offered no advantage over placebo for parent ratings of social functioning or for ratings of parental stress. MPH effects on early academic skills have not been reported for the PATS or any other controlled medication study with this age group.

As is the case for functional impairment, there are virtually no studies examining the impact of stimulant medication over a longer time period than a 1- to 2-month controlled trial. Ninety-five children from the PATS completed a 10-month open-trial phase on their optimal dosage with continued monitoring and adjustment of medication, as necessary. Initial effects of MPH on parent and teacher ratings of ADHD symptoms and social competence were maintained for most of the participants over the 10-month period (Vitiello et al., 2007). Interestingly, an additional 45 children had started the 10-month open-trial phase but discontinued treatment for a variety of reasons, including adverse side effects, behavior worsening, and switching to longer acting stimulants. Also, the mean dosage for those children who completed the 10-month trial increased from approximately 14 milligrams to 20 milligrams per day.

Although more controlled studies of medication need to be conducted with young children with ADHD, results from the extant literature (especially the PATS) lead to several conclusions. First, the acute effects of MPH and other stimulants on ADHD symptoms is similar to those found for older children with statistically and clinically significant reductions in parent and teacher ratings of inattention and hyperactivity–impulsivity for the majority of treated children. Second, the magnitude of obtained effects is lower than that found for older children, although preschoolers with no or one comorbid disorder may exhibit a more robust MPH response. Third, little is known about stimulant effects on academic and social functioning in this age group. This is a significant gap in the literature given that these functional impairments can deleteriously affect preschool performance in this population. Fourth, a significant percentage of children experience adverse side effects that lead parents to discontinue pharmacologic treatment. Significant decreases in height and weight velocity are of particular concern. Finally, it appears that MPH effects on ADHD symptoms maintain across time (e.g., 10 months), but additional studies are needed to examine long-term effects more comprehensively. Thus, the use of stimulant medication in this population must be approached cautiously and must be monitored closely to make treatment decisions that appropriately balance beneficial effects on behavior with the probability of adverse side effects.

## METHODS TO DETERMINE WHETHER MEDICATION IS NECESSARY

Despite the apparent efficacy of stimulant medications in reducing ADHD symptoms in young children, the possible adverse side effects of this treatment as well as the potential success of psychosocial and behavioral interventions warrant conservative use of pharmacotherapy in this age group. Thus, practitioners must use a data-based decision-making approach in guiding families and physicians regarding whether medication treatment is necessary for a specific child with ADHD. The three primary areas to address in this decision-making process are the severity of ADHD symptoms, the degree to which children are impaired in key areas (e.g., development of academic skills, age-appropriate peer relationships), and children's response to behavioral and psychosocial treatments.

One important factor to consider in the medication decision-making process is the severity of ADHD symptomatic behaviors. If difficulties with inattention and hyperactivity–impulsivity are particularly severe, it may be difficult for parents and teachers to implement behavioral procedures as described in earlier chapters. Stated differently, some children may be inattentive, impulsive, or physically active to the degree that it is time-consuming and resource-intensive to modify their behavior simply by manipulating antecedent and consequent events in typical home and preschool settings. In such cases, medication can be tried in concert with behavioral interventions in the hope that a greater response to the latter will result. It is also important to note whether high-severity ADHD symptoms are present across home, preschool, and child care environments. When symptoms are particularly severe and consistent across settings, medication may be helpful in priming child behavior to be responsive to behavioral interventions.

Consideration of symptom severity in making medication decisions must be tempered by several important caveats. First, as discussed in Chapter 1, behaviors symptomatic of ADHD are common in the preschool population, and thus symptom severity must be evaluated using psychometrically sound instruments. Further, the consistency of ADHD behavioral severity across times and settings needs to be considered before concluding that children's symptoms are in the highly severe range. Second, symptom severity should never be discerned solely on the basis of parent and teacher ratings; the practitioner should also directly observe children's behavior in the home, classroom, or both. Direct observation is necessary because adult ratings may be biased or skewed as a function of individual tolerance levels for active behavior as well as experience with children's behavior at a given developmental level. Also, children's disruptive behavior may appear severe because the environment is chaotic, disorganized, and poorly managed. In such cases, changing the environmental structure or moving children out of problematic environments should take place before medication is considered. Finally, in many cases, it is difficult to determine the clinical significance of symptom severity without considering the degree to which symptoms impair children's functioning. Thus, the latter needs to be considered along with symptom severity in making medication decisions.

The degree to which ADHD symptoms impair academic and social functioning is a critical factor to consider when determining whether pharmacotherapy is necessary. Impairment should be assessed using several psychometrically sound measures (as described in Chapter 1) and across home and preschool settings. If children show severe impairment in the development of academic skills or age-appropriate peer relationships, then an evaluation of medication treatment should be considered. Although impairment severity is somewhat difficult to assess, one way to define this is in terms of deviation from age-based norms. Specifically, severe impairment could be defined as a score on a measure of social or academic functioning that is 2 or more standard deviations below the mean for a child's age and gender. Of course, the caveats provided previously must be considered, including the need to ensure that severe impairment is being reported across respondents and settings. It is important to note that behavioral and academic interventions described in prior chapters typically are effective in addressing mild and moderate severity of impairment. If academic or social impairment is consistently reported in the severe range, then an evaluation of medication treatment may be warranted. It should be reiterated, however, that whether medication can result in improvements in academic and social functioning is unclear. Rather, pharmacotherapy may work indirectly, such as by improving attention so that children can benefit from academic instruction. Still, even in such cases, specific social and preacademic interventions are advised along with medication.

Perhaps the most important criterion for considering pharmacotherapy is the degree to which children respond to behavioral interventions. A response-to-intervention approach is useful in determining need for special education services in public school settings (Jimerson, Burns, & VanDerHeyden, 2007). A similar tactic can be used to ascertain whether young children with ADHD may require an intrusive treatment such as psychotropic medication. Specifically, children's response to the early intervention protocol described in Chapters 3 and 4 should be assessed over a reasonable length of time (e.g., several months). Those children who demonstrate little to no change (or regression) following implementation of assessment-based intervention across settings may require medication as an adjunctive treatment. Care should be taken to ensure that parents and teachers have implemented behavioral interventions with sufficient integrity before reaching any conclusions regarding treatment efficacy. Further, a clear definition of treatment response should be used so that accurate decisions are reached. For example, a criterion of 30% reduction in parent and teacher ratings of target behaviors may represent a positive response to treatment, whereas change of less than 10% could indicate a lack of treatment response.

Ultimately, the combination of these three factors (symptom severity, degree of impairment, and response to behavioral intervention) should be used in concert to determine the need for pharmacotherapy. In those cases in which symptoms are sufficiently severe, impairment is clinically significant, and properly implemented behavioral intervention has generated little response, then medication treatment should be evaluated. To the degree that there are discrepancies across these factors, modification of behavioral intervention (e.g., increasing frequency of reinforcement) should be considered before evaluating medication.

## ASSESSMENT OF MEDICATION OUTCOMES

After a decision to prescribe medication is reached, a multimethod, comprehensive assessment of medication response should be used to decide whether this treatment is effective and to determine the optimal dosage. Although many young children with ADHD are likely to respond positively to a CNS stimulant medication, there are individual differences in the degree of response, and effects may vary as a function of dosage. Thus, it is important to use an objective evaluation process that includes multiple measures that are reliable and valid for repeated administration across dosage conditions. Further, explicit criteria should be used to determine the overall efficacy of the medication as well as the dosage that is optimal for enhancing functioning while minimizing adverse side effects. A case example is presented at the end of this section to illustrate the use of the medication evaluation process in making treatment decisions.

## Medication Evaluation Process

On the basis of prior studies of stimulant medication for treating ADHD, a comprehensive medication evaluation should include several key steps (see Exhibit 7.1). First, a treatment team consisting of the parent(s), physician, psychologist (or other mental health professional), and preschool teacher should design the medication trial a priori. Specifically, this team should identify and agree on specific timelines, measures, and procedures that will be used in conducting the evaluation. For example, dosage conditions could be changed on a weekly basis with the psychologist collecting measures of behavioral response in home and preschool settings at the conclusion of each week.

The next step to the medication trial is to identify the key areas of functioning (e.g., academic, social, behavioral) that may change as a function of treatment. Stated differently, the team should decide on the primary targets for medication treatment. Many times, the primary objective is to reduce behaviors that are symptomatic of ADHD, ODD, or both. As emphasized

### EXHIBIT 7.1
#### Important Features of Medication Evaluation Procedures

1. Medication trial is designed through consultation between the practitioner and the prescribing physician.
2. Specific timelines, measures, and procedures are identified and agreed on.
3. Areas of functioning (e.g., cognitive, academic, behavioral) to assess are identified, and measures to document change are used.
4. Data using objective, psychometrically sound measures (e.g., behavior rating scales and direct observations) are collected across dosage conditions.
5. Potential side effects are identified, and measures to assess these are used.
6. Data are collected during both nonmedication and medication conditions in as controlled a fashion as possible.
7. Data are summarized through graphic display, tabular presentation of statistics, or both to facilitate interpretation.
8. Interpretation of outcomes is made collaboratively with the child's physician, and recommendations are clearly communicated to the child's parents.

From *Promoting Children's Health: Integrating Health, School, Family, and Community Systems* (p. 133), by T. J. Power, G. J. DuPaul, E. S. Shapiro, and A. E. Kazak, 2003, New York, NY: Guilford Press. Copyright 2003 by Guilford Press. Adapted with permission.

throughout this text, however, it is also important for treatment to target important areas of functioning in addition to symptoms. In any case, after targets are agreed on, then measures to assess areas of functioning are identified (see the Medication Evaluation Measures section in this chapter). These objective, psychometrically sound measures (e.g., behavior rating scales, direct observations) are collected across dosage conditions to document medication-induced change.

In similar fashion, potential adverse side effects (e.g., insomnia, reduction in appetite) are identified, and measures to assess these side effects are used. Typically, parents and teachers are asked to complete brief ratings of the presence and severity of side effects. For example, Barkley and Murphy (2006) provided a brief rating of stimulant side effects that is useful for repeated assessment across dosage conditions. These ratings should be collected on the same schedule as the primary outcome measures.

After the timing and measurement decisions are made, data are collected across several dosage conditions, including at least one period of nonmedication. The inclusion of a nonmedication phase is critical in evaluating the degree to which medication leads to changes that are clinically significant improvements relative to times when medication is absent. In empirical studies, placebo controls are used because these not only help to gauge functioning during nonmedication conditions but also control for potential confounding variables such as expectancy effects (i.e., person believing that change has occurred on the basis of knowing that treatment has been received). Of course, the feasibility of using placebo controls in a community setting is typically limited; however, some pharmacies are able to provide placebos when prescribed. The more likely nonmedication condition is simply a period of time when medication is not dispensed. In the case of stimulants, alternating periods of medication and nonmedication is not problematic given their pharmacokinetic properties (e.g., complete elimination by the body within 24 hours). Other medications (e.g., atomoxetine) cannot be abruptly withdrawn, and the physician must design a gradual stepdown to nonmedication.

After the trial is completed, data should be summarized across dosage conditions using either a graphic display of outcomes as a function of dosage (e.g., see Figure 7.1 later in the chapter) or a table of scores across conditions. Pediatricians prefer brief, to-the-point reports of evaluations rather than lengthy reports (Hailemariam, Bradley-Johnson, & Johnson, 2002); thus, the simpler the data presentation, the better. The psychologist is then in a position to offer data-based recommendations to the treatment team regarding the degree to which medication leads to clinical improvement and which dosage appeared to optimize functioning while minimizing adverse side effects (see the Criteria for Decision Making in this chapter). These recommendations must be made in a clear, respectful manner to children's parents and physicians.

## Medication Evaluation Measures

Multiple measures collected across settings should be included in the medication evaluation. The perceptions of key adults (i.e., parents and teachers) should be supplemented with direct observations of child behavior as well as permanent products (e.g., completion of assigned tasks). Measures used in the evaluation should possess several important properties. First, they need to be brief enough to be feasible for repeated administration across days or weeks. Second, measures should have established reliability and validity for evaluating treatment outcome. Specifically, adequate levels of test–retest reliability and criterion-related validity are critical. Further, empirical data demonstrating that a measure is sensitive to the effects of treatment are critical. Finally, measures must address the behaviors or areas of functioning identified as primary targets by the treatment team.

Many of the measures discussed in Chapter 1 are appropriate for evaluating the effects of medication. Specifically, narrowband rating scales of ADHD-related behaviors can be used to document the degree to which medication reduces the frequency and severity of ADHD symptoms. As such, parents and teachers would complete brief questionnaires such as the ADHD Rating Scale—IV—Preschool Version (McGoey et al., 2007) or the ADHD Symptoms Rating Scale (Phillips, Greenson, Collett, & Gimpel, 2002) at the conclusion of each dosage condition (including nonmedication). If problems with noncompliance and aggression are of primary interest, then subscales from the Conners Teacher Rating Scale—Revised for Preschoolers (Purpura & Lonigan, 2009) or the Disruptive Behavior Disorders Rating Scale (Pelham, Gnagy, Greenslade, & Milich, 1992) could be used.

Changes in children's disruptive and inattentive behaviors can also be documented using structured direct observations. Observation codes such as the Early Screening Project coding system (Walker, Severson, & Feil, 1995) and the Classroom Observation Code (Abikoff, Gittelman-Klein, & Klein, 1977) can be used across dosage phases to assess behavioral change during unstructured and structured situations, respectively. If observations are used, care should be taken to collect data during times when the medication is most active. For immediate-release stimulant medications, observations should be conducted approximately 1.5 to 3 hours postingestion. Alternatively, for long-acting or extended-release stimulants, it is best to collect observation data at least 2 hours after ingestion. As much as possible, observations should be conducted under similar conditions during each medication phase. In particular, it is important that time after ingestion and the observed classroom situation are as consistent as possible so that data are not appreciably affected by variables other than medication.

Possible changes in academic and social functioning should also be assessed. Parent and teacher ratings on the Impairment Rating Scale (Fabiano et al., 2006) or the Children's Problem Checklist (Healey, Miller, Castelli, Marks, & Halperin, 2008) can be used to show general changes in impairment as a function of medication. More specific measures of social skills (e.g., Social Skills Improvement Systems; Gresham & Elliott, 2008) or academic skills (e.g., Academic Competence Evaluation Scale; DiPerna & Elliott, 2000) can be used; however, these ratings tend to be rather lengthy and may be unwieldy for repeated, regular administration. Further, it is unlikely that they will reflect change over the course of a short-term medication evaluation. Brief measures of early literacy (e.g., Dynamic Indicators of Basic Early Literacy Skills; Kaminski & Good, 1996) or early numeracy (e.g., Preschool Numeracy Indicators; Floyd, Hojnoski, & Key, 2006; Hojnoski, Silberglitt, & Floyd, 2009) are more feasible and treatment-sensitive measures that should be used whenever possible when medication effects on early academic skills are of interest.

### Criteria for Decision Making

After the medication evaluation is completed, data must be displayed and interpreted to address two overriding clinical decisions. One decision is whether medication is effective in bringing about clinically significant change. The other decision is which dosage, if any, is optimal for improving children's functioning while not leading to significant adverse side effects. Analytic methods typically employed to evaluate data collected in single-subject research designs (Kazdin, 2001) should be used to document medication-induced changes in level and trend across phases. Northup and colleagues (1997, 1999) have conducted several studies showing how single-subject design methods can be used successfully in delineating medication effects for children with ADHD. This analytic methodology requires several data points per phase that may be feasible for some measures (e.g., observations) but not others (e.g., rating scales).

Regardless of the number of data points per phase, practitioners must determine whether clinically significant change has occurred. One methodology that may assist in this decision is using the reliable change index described by Jacobson and Truax (1991). This index takes the standard error of measurement (based on test–retest reliability) of a given measure into account in determining whether reliable change has occurred. Stated differently, the reliable change index indicates when differences in scores across medication phases are not readily accounted for by the limited reliability of the measure and regression to the mean artifacts. The reliable change index has been used successfully in characterizing effects of MPH on the behavioral functioning of children with ADHD (e.g., Rapport et al., 1994).

EXHIBIT 7.2
Using Data to Make Medication Decisions: Questions to Consider When
Interpreting Medication Evaluation Data

1. Do any of the active medication conditions lead to reliable change in the desired direction for a particular measure? Is there an overall medication effect?
2. What is the lowest medication dosage that leads to the greatest reliable change and the fewest adverse side effects? What is the minimally effective dosage?
3. To what degree is there consistency in dose–response across symptoms, behaviors, and measures of functional impairment? What dosage leads to the most consistent effects across measures?

After the practitioner or treatment team has gathered and analyzed the data, three important questions must be answered (Power, DuPaul, Shapiro, & Kazak, 2003; see Exhibit 7.2). First, is there an overall medication effect? The answer to this question is determined by examining whether any of the active medication conditions leads to reliable change in the desired direction for one or more outcome measures. If any single medication condition leads to reliable change for one key measure (relative to nonmedication), then an overall medication effect is present.

The second question is what is the minimally effective dosage (Gadow, 1986)? To address this question, the practitioner or treatment team must first identify those dosage conditions that led to reliable change in the therapeutic direction on each measure. Then, those dosages that also did not lead to an increase in frequency or severity of adverse side effects are highlighted. Finally, the lowest dosage among those remaining is determined to be the minimally effective dosage for each specific measure.

The final question is whether there are consistent results across measures, settings, and respondents. Ideally, the same minimally effective dosage will be found for each measure. Unfortunately, this is rarely the case in actual practice. Thus, the treatment team usually must make a decision based one of two criteria (Power et al., 2003). One option is to choose the dosage based on the medication condition that was most frequently identified as the minimally effective dosage across measures. The other option is to choose the dosage by selecting the condition that was the minimally effective dosage for one or more key target outcomes. In the latter case, the team may prioritize outcomes and select dosage on the basis of relative impact on the most important one or two measures.

## Medication Evaluation Case Example

Brian was a 5-year-old European American boy diagnosed with ADHD—combined type and ODD who was placed in a general education, pre-kindergarten classroom that held half-day sessions 5 days per week. The initial psychological evaluation indicated that Brian's ADHD symptoms were in the severe range because both parent and teacher ratings on the Preschool ADHD Rating Scale—IV placed him more than 2 standard deviations above the mean for his age and gender for both inattention and hyperactivity–impulsivity. Further, evaluation data indicated that social and academic impairment was significant given that he had made minimal progress in basic early literacy and numeracy skills and also had almost no friends at home or school.

Over a 6-month period, Brian's parents and pre-kindergarten teacher implemented assessment-based behavioral interventions as described in Chapters 3 and 4. Unfortunately, despite the fact that interventions were implemented with a reasonable degree of integrity, Brian showed minimal change in parent and teacher ratings of ADHD and ODD symptoms (supported through direct observation data) as well as minimal progress in development of early literacy and numeracy skills. The treatment team (Brian's parents, teacher, school psychologist, and physician) decided that Brian's lack of progress was due to the severity of his inattention and hyperactivity–impulsivity. On that basis, a trial of stimulant medication (MPH) was prescribed as an adjunct to ongoing behavioral intervention.

Three relatively low dosages (5 milligrams, 10 milligrams, and 15 milligrams) of MPH were prescribed. A generic, short-acting compound was initially used because the team's objective was to see whether the medication led to clinical improvements before trying a longer acting and potentially more expensive medication regimen. After 1 week of baseline or no medication, these three active dosage conditions were implemented for 1 week each. Four primary outcome measures were used based on the most important targets for Brian's behavior: total score on the Preschool ADHD Rating Scale—IV (parent), percentage of observation intervals in which off-task behavior was observed in the preschool classroom, item scores for academic impairment (teacher), and social impairment (parent) on the Impairment Rating Scale. In addition, total side effects frequency rating (parent) using the Barkley and Murphy (2006) side effects measure was used to look at adverse side effects.

Results for Brian's medication evaluation are presented for primary measures and side effects in Figures 7.1 and 7.2, respectively. All three active dosages led to a 30% reduction and reliable change (improvement) in parent-reported ADHD symptoms and direct observations of off-task behavior in the preschool classroom. In fact, there was an apparent negative linear dose–response effect, indicating that increasing dosages led to stepwise improvements in ADHD symptoms (see Figure 7.1). Further, two of the three dosages (5 milligrams and 10 milligrams) led to 30% reduction in academic and social impairment ratings. To determine the minimally effective dosage, Brian's treatment team also needed to examine adverse side effects. Parent report of side-effect fre-

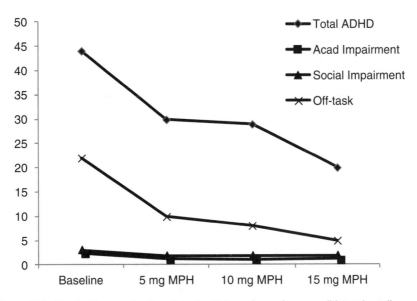

*Figure 7.1.* Medication evaluation data for Brian across four conditions: baseline, 5 milligrams, 10 milligrams, and 15 milligrams methylphenidate (MPH). Data are presented for four primary measures: total score on the Preschool ADHD Rating Scale-IV (parents), percentage of intervals where off-task behavior was observed (direct observation), score on the academic impairment item from the Impairment Rating Scale (teacher), and score on the social impairment item from the Impairment Rating Scale (parent). Acad = academic.

quency actually decreased with the lowest MPH dosage and then systematically increased over baseline levels for the two higher dosages (see Figure 7.2). In looking at the consistency of findings across measures, the team concluded that the 5-milligram MPH dosage was the overall minimally effective dosage and recommended continued treatment at this level of medication.

## CONCLUSIONS

Although psychotropic medication, especially CNS stimulants, is considered a first-line treatment for ADHD in older children and adolescents, pharmacotherapy is a secondary option for treatment of this disorder in young children. Stated differently, psychosocial (primarily behavioral) interventions are the primary treatment choice to address ADHD symptoms in preschool-age children. Several factors support this conclusion. First, controlled studies of stimulant medication in young children have shown small to moderate improvements in symptoms; however, the risk for adverse side effects, including growth inhibition, is higher than that seen for older children.

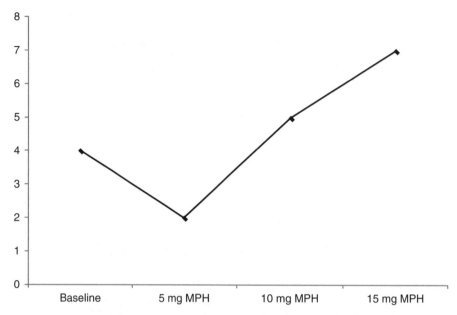

*Figure 7.2.* Total number of adverse side effects reported by Brian's parents as a function of four medication conditions: baseline, 5 milligrams methylphenidate (MPH), 10 milligrams MPH, and 15 milligrams MPH.

Thus, the risk–benefit ratio for this treatment approach may be skewed in the direction of higher risk, thereby precluding the use of medication for many young children. Second, little is known about the long-term benefits and risks of stimulants started at an early age. In particular, almost no data exist regarding the impact of this treatment on early academic skill and social relationship development. Finally, behavioral interventions implemented at home and preschool are efficacious for addressing symptoms and at least some areas of impairment. Further, the behavioral strategies do not carry the risk of adverse side effects seen with medication.

Presumably, the majority of young children with ADHD will be treated exclusively with behavioral and academic interventions; however, some children will require a more intensive treatment because of the severity of their symptoms and impairment, as well as lack of sufficient responsiveness to non-pharmacologic interventions. Thus, stimulant medication should be considered an adjunct to behavioral intervention for those children whose ADHD and associated impairment are severe. It is not clear whether the same recommendation can be made for nonstimulant compounds (e.g., atomoxetine) because no controlled studies of these medications have been published to date. When medication is considered, a data-based decision-making approach should be used to determine whether medication works and which dosage optimizes child functioning. Mental health and educational practitioners should collaborate with families and physicians to make data-based decisions about medication.

To determine whether psychotropic medication could be a first-line treatment option for some young children with ADHD, additional research will be necessary. As mentioned previously, it is critical to determine what impact, if any, stimulants and other compounds have on social and early academic functioning. Although the PATS provided preliminary evidence for a salutary effect on social competence, at least as rated by teachers, more comprehensive assessment of this complex area of functioning is needed. Second, although some long-term studies of stimulants have been conducted with the ADHD population, there are no extant investigations of longitudinal benefits and risks of medication initiated during the preschool years. There may be important differences in outcome when medication is begun during a sensitive period of brain development. Finally, no matter what additional findings are obtained, it is unlikely that medication will be sufficient as a sole treatment for ADHD. Thus, studies examining medication combined with behavioral interventions should be conducted to examine single and combined effects of each treatment modality, as has been done with older children (e.g., MTA Cooperative Group, 1999). As is the case for older children with ADHD (e.g., Fabiano et al., 2007), it may be possible to use a lower dosage of each treatment when stimulants and behavioral strategies are combined.

# 8

# SUPPORT FOR FAMILIES

As we have advocated throughout the previous chapters, parent-implemented intervention should be the first course of treatment for young children showing symptoms of attention-deficit/hyperactivity disorder (ADHD). Home-based intervention is instrumental for improving child outcomes and is particularly effective when implemented early on, when behavior problems are just emerging. The importance of parent-implemented intervention is based on the commonly held belief that environmental factors play a larger role than biological factors in the development of comorbid and potentially more serious disorders commonly associated with ADHD, such as oppositional defiant disorder (ODD) and conduct disorder (CD) (e.g., Barkley, 2006; see also Introduction and Chapter 2, this volume). Specifically, the manner in which parents interact with their children plays a critical role in determining the course of problem behavior (Patterson, 1995). With effective prevention and response strategies, problem behavior is likely to decrease. In the absence of such strategies, problem behaviors may be exacerbated.

Although all parents have the potential to learn strategies and interaction styles that can improve their children's outcomes, several variables may interfere with parents' ability to implement those strategies regularly and consistently. For instance, family stress, parental psychopathology, coping

167

strategies, family dynamics, and social support all play a role in parents' response to their child's behavior challenges (Barkley, 2006). Hence, early interventionists now advocate for a family-oriented focus rather than a child-oriented focus (e.g., Gallimore, Weisner, Kaufman, & Bernheimer, 1989). Specifically, effective child intervention requires a consideration of family challenges, values, priorities, and culture. Understanding the unique situations and needs of families allows practitioners and clinicians to provide the kind of support necessary for child success.

This approach to child intervention has been widely embraced in the field of disabilities and is considered best practice (e.g., Bruder, 2000; Ingber & Dromi, 2010). The approach has been applied broadly, including at the statewide level (e.g., Gallagher, Rhodes, & Darling, 2004). In addition, empirical research suggests that a family-focused approach to early intervention has many beneficial outcomes compared with alternative approaches. For example, Brookman-Frazee and Koegel (2010) compared a clinician-directed parent education model with a parent–clinician partnership model. The parent–clinician partnership model resulted in reduced levels of parent stress and increased levels of parent confidence. Further, levels of positive child affect and increased levels of child engagement were higher when parents participated in the partnership model.

In this chapter, we begin with a discussion of current views toward family support. We then outline the steps for building an effective partnership with families. Subsequently, we describe the variables that can affect intervention implementation by parents. Cultural issues and their consideration when developing intervention plans are discussed next. We conclude with recommendations for working with families.

## CURRENT APPROACHES FOR SUPPORTING FAMILIES

Current approaches for working with families emphasize the importance of a collaborative partnership. This differs from an "expert model" in which the practitioner's role is to impart information to the family. More recently, effective family support has shifted to a reciprocal relationship in which practitioners and family members mutually contribute to intervention development. This partnership leads to interventions that offer a good ecological fit for families and their home environments. Such interventions are consistent with family values, accommodate family challenges, reflect family culture, and fit within family routines.

A collaborative partnership with a family means that professionals and family members have a relationship in which roles are agreed on and common goals have been established (Dunst & Paget, 1991). As defined by

Lucyshyn, Horner, Dunlap, Albin, and Ben (2002), family–professional collaboration requires a respectful, trusting, and caring relationship in which there is an equal partnership. This relationship allows both parents and professionals to exchange ideas, make recommendations, and address concerns.

Collaborative partnerships capitalize on the contributions of both professionals and family members. Professionals may be "experts" in specific intervention procedures, but parents are "experts" in their own child. The role of the professional is to ensure that parents have the specific skills and strategies to address their child's behavior problems (Koegel, Koegel, Boettcher, & Brookman-Frazee, 2005). Family members have detailed knowledge about their children, including their strengths, needs, preferences, skills, and other information critical for an effective intervention plan (Turnbull & Turnbull, 2000). Further, families can share information about their goals, values, routines, resources, and culture that are necessary considerations for an effective intervention (Lucyshyn & Albin, 1993).

## DEVELOPING A PARTNERSHIP WITH FAMILIES

Establishing a collaborative partnership with families is an ongoing process of open communication and feedback (Lucyshyn & Albin, 1993). Koegel, Koegel, Boettcher, and Brookman-Frazee (2005) delineated four important considerations for developing a collaborative relationship (see Table 8.1, which is based on guidelines provided by Koegel et al., 2005). The first is to establish an alliance with the family. This involves ensuring that professionals offer a good match for the family. For example, when professionals are either matched or familiar with the cultural and linguistic backgrounds of a family, communication and understanding are facilitated. This enhanced communication and understanding can result in an intervention plan that offers a good fit for the family. Also, some families prefer to work with male or female professionals. This gender match can ease the partnership development. Finally, family members may respond to certain personality types, such as supportive, animated, or directive. When professionals and parents are well matched, the intervention plan and ongoing support are likely to be more effective. When exact matches are not possible, practitioners must gain an understanding of family preferences and beliefs (e.g., cultural values, favored interaction style) and make adjustments to their usual professional style. If practitioners are unable to modify their style to meet a family's needs, and better matches are unavailable, the family should be referred elsewhere.

The second consideration is to gain an understanding of the family's priorities. Professionals and parents may view and/or prioritize a child's behavior problems very differently. Research indicates that interventions focused

## TABLE 8.1
### Strategies for Developing a Collaborative Relationship With Families

| Goal | Process | Considerations |
|------|---------|----------------|
| Establish an alliance with the family | Match professional to family | Cultural and linguistic similarities<br>Gender preference<br>Personality type |
| Understand family priorities | Mutually identify goals | Harmful and dangerous behaviors<br>Behaviors stressful to family<br>Long-term consequences |
| Determine fit of intervention with family routine | Understand family daily activities | Competing parent responsibilities<br>Needs of all family members |
| Understand family culture | Become familiar with family values | Expectations of children<br>Parenting approaches<br>Expectations of professionals |
| Determine family strengths | Identify how strengths of family members can assist intervention process | Family support networks<br>Skill at implementing intervention |

From *Designing Positive Behavior Supports for Students* (pp. 340–344), by L. M. Bambara and L. Kern (Eds.), 2005, New York, NY: Guilford Press. Copyright 2005 by Guilford Press. Adapted with permission.

on goals that family members do not view as important are not implemented or maintained over time (Steibel, 1999). Hence, it is important that goals are mutually identified and agreed on. In the case of young children with symptoms of ADHD, this may involve extensive discussion about the progression of ADHD so that families appreciate the need to prevent more serious problems. At the same time, certain child behaviors (e.g., high levels of activity) may be stressful to families but do not cause immediate harm or danger. These might be identified as a priority for a family and should be simultaneously addressed along with other more serious problem behaviors.

The third consideration is the extent to which the intervention plan can be incorporated into the family routine. It is difficult for families to maintain an intervention that requires extreme deviations to their ongoing routines. Professionals must understand a family's daily activities, including the needs and demands of multiple children, to develop and refine a plan that can and will be readily implemented over time.

The degree to which the professional understands the family's culture is a fourth consideration. Many intervention programs have been developed for and evaluated with families of European American background. The appropriateness of such programs with families from diverse ethnic and cultural backgrounds needs to be carefully considered. Further, families from different cultural backgrounds have diverse values, expectations for their children, and parenting approaches. This diversity also may extend to a family's willingness to accept professional services for their child. Effective family intervention requires fully understanding the cultural perspectives and values of each family. The history and traditions of a family's culture can be easily found on the Internet. In addition, several organizations focus on providing technical assistance to promote equity, access, and participation, such as the National Center for Culturally Responsive Education Systems (http://www.nccrest.org) and the Equity Alliance at Arizona State University (http://www.equity allianceatasu.org). Finally, numerous publications are geared toward helping practitioners develop an understanding of family cultural differences (e.g., Harry, 2002; Heffron, Grunstein, & Tilmon, 2007; Hepburn, 2006; Lynch & Hanson, 2004; Sylva, 2005).

A final consideration is the extent to which the family's strengths have been assessed. Strengths within a family provide opportunities that can enhance intervention efforts. For example, if families have strong support networks, they can solicit assistance and support in times of stress. Similarly, if one family member is able to implement interventions consistently, he or she can serve as a coach to others who have more difficulty.

## VARIABLES AFFECTING PARENTS AND CARE PROVIDERS AND CHILD OUTCOMES

When working with families, it is important to understand the multiple variables that may play a role in parents' ability to implement interventions effectively (see Table 8.2). Intervention can be improved by understanding the complexities of family life and the specific ways that variables influence intervention implementation for each particular family. These variables include parent stress, parent–child interactions, parent psychopathology, acceptance of disability by family members, culture and child-rearing practices, as well as social support and empowerment.

### Parent Stress

One major variable that affects every parent's ability to interact productively with their child and address behavioral issues is parent stress. In the case of parenting a child with a disability, the presence of the disability alone accounts for a significant amount of added stress (Neely-Barnes & Dia, 2008).

TABLE 8.2
Variables That Affect Care Providers and Potential Consequences

| Variable | Potential consequences |
| --- | --- |
| Parent stress | Difficulty managing child problem behavior |
| | Problems with attachment (fathers) |
| | Collateral mental health problems |
| Ineffective parent–child interactions | Increased child problem behaviors |
| | Negative and directive parenting style |
| | Noncompliant child behavior across settings |
| Parent psychopathology | Development of child conduct disorders |
| Failure to accept disability | Rejection of services |
| | Limited participation in interventions |
| Culture | Use of "traditional" parenting approaches |
| | Involvement of multiple care providers |
| | Range of openness to information sharing |
| | Preference for differing types of communication |
| Lack of social support | Increased parent stress |
| | Poor quality of life |
| | Limited feelings of parent empowerment |

Specifically, comparative research studies have shown that parents (particularly mothers) of children with disabilities experience a significantly higher level of stress than parents without disabilities (e.g., Baker-Ericzén, Brookman-Frazee, & Stahmer, 2005; Dyson, 1997; Mash & Johnston, 1983). However, research further suggests that problem behavior, which may be more common with particular disabilities (e.g., ADHD), is the actual source of stress, rather than the disability itself (e.g., Baker, Blacher, & Olsson, 2005).

In the case of parents of children with ADHD, research has isolated a number of specific problems that cause parents a large amount of stress. In a study of mothers of 104 children with ADHD, Anastopoulos, Guevremont, Shelton, and DuPaul (1992) found that child aggression, severity of ADHD symptoms, and child health accounted for 43% of the variance in parenting stress. Although much of the research regarding stress has been conducted with mothers, research indicates fathers of children with ADHD also experience significant stress, but it may emerge in different forms. For example, Baker et al. (2005) found that fathers of children with ADHD report difficulties in feeling attached to their child.

Child problem behavior and parent stress also have been associated with self-reports of poor parenting efficacy (Kersh, Hedvat, Hauser-Cram, & Warfield, 2006), poor parental mental health (Herring et al., 2006), and marital problems (Simmerman, Blacher, & Baker, 2001). Hence, these problems contribute to myriad parenting and family challenges. At the same time, this research has important implications for interventionists. Specifically, reducing child problem behavior may lead to reductions in parental stress and related problems.

### Parent–Child Interactions

Another variable that has a large impact on child outcomes is parent–child interactions. A number of interactions and parental responses appear unique to children with ADHD. That is, certain parent–child interactions occur far more often in families with children with ADHD and are specific to children with ADHD and not their siblings (e.g., Danforth, Barkley, & Stokes, 1991). One is a coercive interaction style (Patterson, Reid, & Dishion, 1992). Coercive interactions follow a specific course that begins with problem behavior exhibited by the child, generally in the context of a demand (e.g., "Put your toys away"). The child's problem behavior commonly takes the form of noncompliance, tantrums, crying, or aggression. In response to the problem behavior, the parent withdraws the demand in an effort to stop the problem behavior. Withdrawing the demand inadvertently teaches the child that problem behavior is an effective means of avoiding demands and controlling the immediate situation. Eventually, the child generalizes the use of problem behaviors to control other types of situations, such as peer interactions in the preschool settings. The difficulties that parents experience in following through with instructions and setting limits most likely result from the frequency and persistence of problem behaviors exhibited by children with ADHD.

In similar fashion, parents may react to children's tantrums or noncompliance by using upper limit controls (e.g., yelling, threatening punishment, spanking). In some cases, children may comply or give in to parental demands when upper limit controls are used. When this happens, parental use of threats, yelling, and physical punishment is reinforced or rewarded by the child's capitulation. Therefore, in subsequent negative interactions, parents may be more likely to use upper limit controls that can sometimes lead to short-term improvement in child behavior but are rarely effective over the long term. Thus, parent education must focus on improving parenting responses when children exhibit problem behaviors and reducing these coercive exchanges.

In addition, parents tend to be more directive with children with ADHD, such as issuing high rates of demands, and are less likely to reward positive behavior (Danforth et al., 1991; DuPaul et al., 2001). They also may be more emotional with a child with ADHD, outwardly displaying anger and resentment (e.g., Buhrmester, Camparo, Christensen, Gonzales, & Hinshaw, 1992; Taylor, Sandberg, Thorley, & Giles, 1991). Further, in the presence of both parents, mother–child conflicts may result in an increase in father–child conflicts as well (e.g., Buhrmester et al., 1992). Research has shown that these problematic parent–child interactions predict noncompliance in school and other settings, as well as other problem behaviors in the home (e.g., Anderson, Hinshaw, & Simmel, 1994). Thus, intervention to improve parent–child interactions may result in generalized behavior reductions across settings.

## Parent Psychopathology

As described previously, the challenging behavior frequently exhibited by young children with ADHD sets an interactive cycle in motion in which negative parental reactions further exacerbate the child's problems. Although this negative interactive cycle may be specific to the child with ADHD, parental psychopathology is also a risk factor that may contribute to the development of more severe child conduct problems (Johnston & Mash, 2001). ADHD is highly heritable; however, the research suggests that having a parent with ADHD alone only slightly increases the risk of a child developing comorbid ODD or CD (Lahey et al., 1988). Rather, it is the presence of comorbid ODD, CD, or antisocial personality disorder in a parent that greatly increases the risk of a child developing a similar comorbid disorder. For instance, Faraone, Biederman, Jetton, and Tsuang (1997) found that 46% of children with ADHD and comorbid ODD had parents with ADHD and comorbid ODD, CD, or antisocial personality disorder.

Of particular importance to practitioners and clinicians is the manner in which characteristics that are associated with psychiatric disorders manifest in parent–child interactions. Nigg and Hinshaw (1998) found that children with ADHD and ODD or CD have parents with personality traits that are significantly different from parents of control children. Specifically, fathers of children with comorbidities show lower levels of agreeableness, greater levels of neuroticism, and a more frequent incidence of generalized anxiety disorder, whereas mothers also show greater levels of neuroticism as well as lower conscientiousness and greater incidence of depression.

Maternal depression has been extensively studied, particularly in relation to the development of conduct problems in children (Cummings & Davies, 1999; Downey & Coyne, 1990; Elgar, McGrath, & Waschbusch, 2004). Research has found a strong association between maternal depression and both internalizing and externalizing behavior problems, with children of depressed mothers having diagnosable psychiatric problems at 3 to 4 times the rate of nondepressed mothers (Anderson & Hammen, 1993; Cummings & Davies, 1999). It appears that there is a bidirectional influence of negative maternal behaviors and child problem behaviors. Specifically, depressed mothers tend to exhibit more negative, critical, hostile, unengaged, and nonsupportive behaviors when interacting with their children, and these behaviors are exacerbated by child problem behavior (e.g., Burge & Hammen,

1991; Hammen, Burge, & Stansbury, 1990). It appears that these influences may be most salient during the early childhood and preschool years (Luthar & Zelazo, 2003), which underscores the importance of early intervention. At the same time, recent research unfortunately suggests that although both maternal depression and parenting behaviors contribute to child conduct problems, parenting behaviors do not completely mediate the effect of maternal depression on child outcomes (Chronis et al., 2007). Hence, although it is critical to improve parent–child interactions, additional protective factors must also be enlisted in families with psychopathology.

### Acceptance of Disability

The reactions of family members to having a child with a disability vary widely. When parents receive a diagnosis of their child's disability, they may experience significant stress and concern about the future (e.g., Koegel, Koegel, Boettcher, & Brookman-Frazee, 2005). These feelings are often more intense when the child exhibits severe symptoms (e.g., Singer & Irvin, 1991).

A family's cultural background also may play a role in parental responses to disability. For example, some families believe that a child's disability is a natural part of life and tend to reject any type of intervention. Other families may reject intervention and services because their culture feels that a child's disability is punishment from God (Chan, 1990; Groce & Zola, 1993). Still other cultures believe that a disability is the result of misdeeds by the pregnant woman or the child in a former life (Chen, Downing, & Peckham-Hardin, 2002). These diverse beliefs may influence a family's effort to seek and accept services.

Further, mothers and fathers may have different reactions to a disability label. In particular, Singh (2003) found that many fathers could be classified as "reluctant believers" or "tolerant nonbelievers" regarding their child's diagnosis of ADHD. In addition, Singh found that fathers were more resistant to accepting a medical framework for their child's diagnosis and more likely to oppose pharmacological intervention than were mothers.

Parental attitudes toward disability have several implications. First, parents who are unwilling to accept their child's disability may be less inclined to become involved in intervention. For example, Singh (2003) suggested that fathers' reluctance toward an ADHD diagnosis may explain their absence in clinical evaluations and research participation. In addition, negative attitudes toward their child's disability may interfere with parenting effectiveness, whereas positive attitudes may enhance child outcomes. Specifically, Lustig (2002) found that families who were able to view their child's disability in a positive manner perceived themselves as more competent and were better adjusted as a family. Similarly, mothers with a more positive perception of their child with a disability tended to rate their family functioning higher (Weinger, 1999). This research suggests the importance of understanding parental attitudes toward their child with ADHD.

## Culture and Child-Rearing Practices

As we noted earlier, a family's cultural background may influence their attitude toward their child with a disability. In addition, a family's culture generally plays a role in their child-rearing practices. That is, families often rely on culture and tradition to guide the manner in which they raise their children. In fact, a study comparing acculturated Mexican American mothers with nonacculturated Mexican American mothers showed that they were more similar to one another with respect to their child-rearing beliefs than to American mothers (Arcia, Reyes-Blanes, & Vazquez-Montilla, 2000).

Cultural approaches to parenting differ greatly. For example, traditional Latino families do not emphasize independence in their children; hence, preschoolers may have limited self-help skills. For families of children with ADHD, this means parents may not readily embrace early skill instruction programs. Further, cultural approaches to child discipline differ greatly. For example, some African American, Asian, and Latino families may use forms of discipline such as spanking, yelling, and shaming their children that diverge from practices typically used in school settings. It is important for practitioners to understand the type of child-rearing practices a family uses. This may play a role in a child's responsiveness to certain forms of discipline applied in schools. Also, parents may be reluctant to use particular practices to which they are unaccustomed. In addition, it is equally important to orient families to American school culture and policies regarding child expectations, learning, and disciplinary procedures (Neely-Barnes & Dia, 2008).

With respect to parenting style, individuals involved in raising a child may differ across families. In many cultures, such as Native American, extended family members play a large role in child rearing (Joe & Malach, 1998). This has implications for who should participate in parent education. Family support may focus on ensuring that all family members who spend time with the child use consistent approaches to reduce behavior problems.

Finally, communication styles may differ across cultures. Differences in communication styles may affect how practitioners develop interventions with families (Correa, 1987). For example, some families from Hispanic, Native American, or Asian backgrounds may be reluctant to openly share information about their family (Harry, 1992). Also, some parents may feel the need to consult family members before making a decision about interventions or services. Thus, it is important for practitioners to solicit information about a family's preferred way of communicating, including when and where visits take place, the pace at which the relationship should be allowed to develop, and the extended family members who should participate in meetings and decision making.

### Social Support and Empowerment

Social support and family empowerment also influence family members' ability to deal effectively with their child's behavior problems. There are many social supports that help families cope with the challenges of having a child with behavior problems (Lucyshyn, Horner, Dunlap, Albin, & Ben, 2002). Informal supports can be offered in the form of assistance with child care and other responsibilities from siblings, grandparents, and other family members. In addition, parents who share similar challenges with their children also can offer support and guidance to one another. Formal supports include services such as speech-language therapy, in-home behavior support, early intervention services, and respite care.

In addition, it is important to consider how social support contributes to family quality of life (Schippers & van Boheemen, 2009). Many families are reluctant to participate in community activities with their child who engages in severe behavior problems. Family members may fail to partake in activities that once provided support and enjoyment, such as going to church or even walking in the park. As families withdraw from pleasurable activities, they begin to feel isolated and powerless. It is important to help families make arrangements so that they can participate in activities they enjoy. This may involve planning regular respite or child care. In addition, it is helpful to inform community members of a child's disability and related behaviors that might be expected. Children are frequently excluded from community settings because people do not understand behavioral differences associated with disabilities and do not have effective strategies to prevent problems. Thus, interventions can be developed for community settings, and community members can be taught to implement those interventions. For example, a Sunday school teacher can be coached through implementation of a plan that calls for frequent breaks, high rates of reinforcement, and token allocation for intervals of appropriate behavior.

A related element of social support is parent empowerment. *Parent empowerment* refers to a parent's ability to participate in and effectively manage interventions and services for their child (Turnbull & Turnbull, 2000). Empowered parents report feeling that they can effectively manage their child's behavior within the context of ongoing routines. In addition, they are able to communicate and negotiate well with preschool staff and other service providers. On the other hand, parents who do not feel empowered report feeling helpless, stressed, and sometimes depressed (Koegel et al., 2005).

Further, they tend to rely extensively on professionals and are unable to see themselves as partners with valuable contributions. Research suggests that the children of families who report feeling empowered make larger improvements than children whose parents do not feel empowered. Hence, practitioners often make family empowerment a goal of intervention (Koegel, Koegel, & Schreibman, 1991).

## RECOMMENDATIONS FOR FAMILY SUPPORT

### Reduce Child Behavior Problems

Perhaps the most important area to address when providing support to families is child behavior problems. As we have discussed, child problem behaviors contribute significantly to parent stress, which in turn interferes with effective parenting. In addition, child problem behaviors often limit a family's community activities and their participation in enjoyable events. This may increase feelings of isolation and further decrease the availability of support.

In addition to the negative influence on parent stress and lifestyle, research suggests that parents often are unable to respond to problem behavior in a way that effectively reduces further occurrences. In fact, their responses may inadvertently aggravate behavior problems. Therefore, it is important to introduce strategies that family members can implement both to prevent problem behavior and to address it effectively when it occurs. As we described in Chapter 3, a behavior plan that includes strategies to reduce child problem behavior also should include strategies to teach appropriate behavior. When prompted and reinforced, these newly learned appropriate behaviors are likely to generalize across settings, allowing the family to feel comfortable participating in fulfilling community activities.

### Improve Parent–Child Interactions

Improving parent–child interactions also should be a goal of family support. It is important not only to improve parent–child interactions that occur in the context of child problem behavior but also to address more general interactions. In particular, we described the manner in which parent psychopathology (i.e., ODD, CD, antisocial personality disorder, depression) is associated with poor child outcomes. Further, we explained the way that certain disorders may manifest during parent–child interactions. For example, mothers experiencing depression tend to be negative, critical, and hostile toward their children (e.g., Burge & Hammen, 1991; Hammen et al., 1990), which can contribute to the development of child

ODD or CD. These problematic interactions appear to be most prominent when children are young (Luthar & Zelazo, 2003). Hence, assisting parents to focus on and reward positive child behaviors early on may partially ameliorate the effect of parent psychopathology. In addition, if parents are not already receiving treatment for their psychopathology, then practitioners should refer parents to appropriate clinicians and support them in seeking treatment.

### Understand Family Culture and Values

Providing effective family support requires understanding family culture and values. Practitioners can work most effectively with families when they understand the many dimensions of culture, particularly those relevant to child rearing. This includes their perspectives on disability, expectations of appropriate behavior, and approach to discipline. In addition, practitioners must understand parents' preferred interaction style and comfort with sharing personal information.

Becoming familiar with each family's values and preferences is a process that may take many weeks, but it establishes the foundation for future positive interactions. At the initiation of services, it is critical to ascertain each family's concerns and priorities for intervention, as well as their expectations. For instance, it is important to identify where problems occur most frequently (including community settings) and make sure that interventions are applicable across settings. In addition, understanding their typical child-rearing practices will assist with developing intervention and compromising, if necessary. Further, it is helpful to determine the style, mode, and frequency of communication that the family believes will be most beneficial. If a family is uncomfortable having practitioners observe during particular family routines, it may be possible to arrange alternative methods to collect assessment information and determine whether intervention is effective. For example, parents may be willing to videotape themselves and their child or collect their own data. Similarly, practitioners can observe family members implementing interventions in alternative settings, making recommendations for generalizing the intervention. Finally, assessing the role of each family member, including extended family, will ensure that all individuals who interact with the child are able to implement the interventions and supports consistently and comfortably.

### Empower the Family

A final recommendation is to encourage family members to take an active role in their child's intervention and the provision of services. This involves first viewing parents as partners who have expertise that is critical to intervention development. It should be clear to parents that they are viewed as collaborators and partners.

In addition, parents should be taught ways to advocate successfully for needed services for their child (Jensen, 2004). Parents who learn advocacy skills when their children are very young are able to improve the likelihood that their children receive beneficial services throughout their educational career, in addition to accessing available community resources. Practitioners should ensure that parents understand the educational services in which their children are entitled under the Individuals With Disabilities Education Improvement Act of 2004, including those available before school entry. Also, parents should have knowledge of Section 504 of the Rehabilitation Act, which provides accommodations to individuals with special needs who do not require special education services. Parents should fully understand the services their child needs, how to ensure the services are provided as designed, and how to assess whether the services are effective.

In addition to school-based services, empowered parents are able to identify and obtain community resources. Practitioners can assist families to understand the questions that are important to ask and how to assert their rights to obtain services to which they are entitled. Further, parents should learn ways to evaluate services objectively and, when judged ineffective or insufficient, to request alternative services.

Beyond school and community services, practitioners can assist parents to work with pediatricians and psychiatrists. This is particularly important for parents of children with ADHD, given the frequent administration of medication with this population. Generally, pediatricians and psychiatrists see children only briefly at scheduled appointments. Thus, they rely extensively on parents for information to determine whether medications are needed or, when prescribed, are effective. When parents have the skills to advocate effectively, their children are more likely to receive appropriate and effective pharmacologic interventions. For an overview of recommendations, see Table 8.3.

## FAMILY SUPPORT CASE EXAMPLE

The Silva family sought intervention services through our project for their 5-year-old grandchild, Ramona, who was identified as having ADHD. Ramona's mother was unable to care for her, so the grandparents assumed parenting responsibilities. The Silvas attended parent education classes, but Ramona continued to engage in problem behaviors. Thus, Tier 2 intervention (i.e., home-based coaching) was initiated. To identify goals that were mutually

TABLE 8.3
Recommendations for Family Support and Implications

| Recommendation | Implications |
|---|---|
| Reduce child problem behaviors | Reductions in parent stress |
| | Increased engagement in community activities |
| Improve parent–child interactions | Decreases in child problem behaviors |
| | Prevention of child conduct problems |
| Appreciate family culture and values | Enhanced family–practitioner relationship |
| | Intervention matched to family preferences |
| | Improved parent adherence to intervention |
| Empower family | Increased feelings of parent efficacy |
| | Improved skill at accessing services |

agreed on, our consultant began by asking the grandparents to develop a list of intervention goals for Ramona. The consultant then reviewed the goals with the grandparents, and they jointly agreed on how the goals would be prioritized. The next objective was for the consultant to understand naturally occurring parent–child interactions as well as regular routines in the home. The consultant spent time observing the family members, also questioning them about procedures and events to understand their culture and values.

The consultant noted that the grandparents were skilled at implementing the interventions they learned during parent education sessions; however, they became tired in the evening hours, and rather than arguing and fighting with Ramona, they gave in to her demands. When the consultant discussed this observation with the Silvas, they agreed that it was difficult to be consistent when they were tired toward the end of the day. Thus, the consultant worked with the Silvas to develop an intervention plan that consisted of predictable schedule for Ramona that included limiting the length of certain activities (television, computer time), scheduling nonpreferred activities before preferred activities (picking up toys before watching television), establishing a consistent bedtime and routines around bedtime. In addition, Ramona's grandparents suggested that they alternate supervision so that each could have scheduled and predictable breaks. Finally, because the Silvas were committed and invested in Ramona's well-being, the consultant suggested they spend time acknowledging each other's strengths and supporting each other. For several sessions, the consultant coached the grandparents through implementation of the schedule, including following through when Ramona resisted.

After 3 weeks of intervention, the Silvas reported substantial improvement in Ramona's behavior. They indicated that the routines were helpful to both Ramona and them. They also stated that alternating primary supervision responsibilities helped them to "get a second wind" and deal more consistently with her. Finally, they noted that verbally discussing their strengths helped them to feel effective and empowered. The consultant continued to work with the Silvas to make minor adjustments to the plan to improve the fit with their routines and preferences.

## CONCLUSIONS

Interventions implemented by family members in the home are critical for preventing serious behavior disorders (e.g., ODD, CD) among children who exhibit symptoms of ADHD. Successful intervention requires that parents implement strategies to prevent problem behaviors from occurring and, when they do occur, respond in ways that reduce the likelihood of reoccurrence. Parents regularly experience challenges that may interfere with their ability to implement successful behavior reduction strategies. Further, the cultural background and values of families play a role in determining the type of interventions they are comfortable implementing. Hence, home-based intervention must take a family-centered focus. This requires that practitioners fully understand each family's culture and values, as well as the variables that may influence intervention implementation. Common challenges and potential solutions are shown in Exhibit 8.1.

When developing a working relationship with families, practitioners must understand the unique contribution that family members offer toward developing an intervention plan. Parents have unique knowledge of their child's history and current behavior problems. Further, a family's culture and personal values should shape the intervention plan. As such, parents should be viewed as collaborative partners in the intervention development process. When parents are treated as important and valued participants, they are able to trust and work productively with practitioners.

Several family variables have been identified that influence the success of a behavior plan. Parent stress is common among parents of children with disabilities and can interfere with effective plan implementation. In addition, parent–child interactions can reduce or exacerbate child problem behavior. Child outcomes may also be affected by the presence of parent psychopathology. Families also have differing attitudes toward having a child with a disability. Further, child-rearing practices vary greatly and may be influenced by culture and tradition. Finally, social support and empowerment can enhance personal feelings of efficacy and success, as well as improve child outcomes.

We recommend several practices that can improve the relationship between practitioners and family members as well as child outcomes. Developing strategies to successfully reduce child behavior problems may be most important because such strategies have many collateral effects, including reducing parent stress and permitting greater engagement in community

## EXHIBIT 8.1
### Challenges to Implementation

*Issue: I am trying to work with a family, but they expect me to tell them what to do and seem to get annoyed when I continually request their input.*

Potential solution: Most families are not accustomed to a professional working collaboratively with them and may have had prior experiences in which their opinions are not valued. At the same time, parents may be frustrated with their child's problem behavior and want solutions. It is important for consultants or clinicians to focus on teaching parents techniques (e.g., scheduled attention, ignoring, praise) but to work collaboratively with parents in choosing how the techniques can be applied. Also, it is important to explain to parents that this type of collaboration is critical so that the techniques are implemented in a way that is acceptable and feasible.

*Issue: Many of the parents in my parent education class are frustrated and stressed and have adopted the opinion that nothing works.*

Potential solution: Many parents have tried endlessly to stop their child's behavior problems to no avail. In these cases, it is important to teach a single technique, rather than overwhelming parents with numerous strategies, and ensure they are able to consistently implement that technique. It helps to collect data so that parents can see their child's improvement, even if it might be slow. Also, parents should understand that the techniques they used with their children without ADHD (e.g., time out) may not necessarily be effective with their child with ADHD. Finally, parent groups, such as parent education classes, can help parents support and encourage one another.

*Issue: I am working with a family that does not trust professionals. They have had bad experiences in the past and are reluctant to open up.*

Potential solution: When parents are distrustful of professionals, it is important to proceed slowly. Parents must fully understand that you are committed to working collaboratively to address their child's behavior issues and are not interested in assigning blame. Parents often report that they are contacted by professionals (e.g., preschool teachers) only when their child misbehaves. For this reason, a strengths-based approach is important. When the strengths of a child (and his or her parents) are capitalized on, parents feel empowered and do not feel blamed for their child's problems.

activities. This involves improving parent–child interactions, both within and outside the context of problem behavior. In addition, at the initiation of intervention, it is important to determine each family's concerns, priorities, and expectations. Practitioners must also determine which communication style and mode are most effective with each particular family. This involves fully understanding a family's culture and values. Finally, a goal of intervention should be to empower families so that they feel confident addressing their child's behavior problems, understand their child's legal rights to services, are able to advocate successfully for their child to obtain school-based and community interventions and services, and can objectively evaluate the effectiveness of each child intervention.

# 9

# FINDINGS AND FUTURE DIRECTIONS

The early intervention approach described in this book is based on empirical investigations conducted by our research team and other investigators interested in young children with attention-deficit/hyperactivity disorder (ADHD) and related disorders. The purpose of this chapter is to present findings regarding the efficacy of early intervention for this population, particularly the results from an ongoing large-scale investigation under our direction. Further, we describe the big ideas underlying this early intervention program as a way of highlighting the major themes of this book. Finally, we discuss future directions for research and practice in early intervention for young children with ADHD.

## EARLY INTERVENTION OUTCOME STUDIES

Over the past few decades, empirical studies have examined the effects of various interventions for young children with or at risk for ADHD. These studies have focused primarily on stimulant medication and behavioral interventions implemented in home or preschool settings (for a review, see Ghuman, Arnold, & Anthony, 2008). Findings from these studies indicate that medication and behavioral interventions significantly reduce sympto-matic behaviors that constitute ADHD and also improve compliance with authority figure commands and classroom rules. For the most part, extant studies have investigated treatment approaches in isolation as opposed to combined treatment protocols applied across settings. In an effort to develop a more comprehensive, cross-setting approach to early intervention, our research team has conducted a series of studies that build toward an integrated, tiered approach in home and preschool settings.

## Early Intervention for ADHD Project

Our investigative team at Lehigh University has conducted several stud-ies that serve as the foundation for the early intervention program described in this book. First, we conducted a pilot investigation of a community-based inter-vention program for young children with ADHD (McGoey et al., 2005). A sample of 57 children (3 and 4 years old) identified as at risk for ADHD were referred by community service providers (e.g., pediatricians), preschool teach-ers, and parents. Children were randomly assigned to a combined intervention group (parent education and preschool behavioral consultation) or to a com-munity treatment control group (families obtained services available in the community, e.g., medication treatment). Dependent measures were collected periodically over a 15-month period and included parent and teacher behavior ratings, observations of parent–child interactions and preschool behavior, doc-umentation of injury rates and medical utilization, parent ratings of stress and family functioning, and a brief test of children's cognitive development. Over the course of the study, the combined intervention group showed improve-ments in child behavior (at home and at school), reductions in parental stress, and more adaptive family coping relative to community treatment controls (McGoey et al., 2005). The primary effect of the combined intervention was to alter the trajectory of child behavior over time relative to the community control participants. Parents and teachers uniformly reported the combined intervention procedures to be highly acceptable and moderately effective. Although few children who received early intervention were placed on psychotropic medication, statistically significant changes in medical use and cognitive development were not obtained in this pilot investigation.

Following this pilot study, we designed a more extensive early interven-tion protocol and evaluated this program in a large sample of young children with ADHD. The purpose of the Early Intervention for ADHD (EIA) project was to evaluate two types of interventions to reduce ADHD-related problem behaviors and, hence, the negative sequelae that typically follow. It is impor-tant to note that for comparative purposes, the participant inclusion criteria for the EIA project were highly similar to the entry criteria for the Preschool

ADHD Treatment Study (PATS; Greenhill et al., 2006), which examined the effects of psychostimulant medication (see Chapter 7, this volume). A multiphase screening process was conducted wherein children were identified as meeting *Diagnostic and Statistical Manual of Mental Disorders* (4th ed., text revision; *DSM–IV–TR*; American Psychiatric Association, 2000) criteria for one of three subtypes of ADHD based on parent diagnostic interviews as well as parent and teacher ratings of ADHD symptoms exceeding the 93rd percentile on the Conners Rating Scales (Conners, 1997). Children with autism, low cognitive ability, or conduct disorder (CD) were excluded. Most (76%) of the sample met criteria for oppositional defiant disorder (ODD).

After screening, 137 children met inclusion criteria. Using a randomized design, children were assigned to either a Multicomponent Intervention Group (MCI) group (*n* = 73) or a Parent Education (PE) group (*n* = 64). No significant group differences in child age, gender, parent occupation, parent education, ADHD subtype, presence of ODD, or receipt of psychotropic medication were indicated by *t* tests or chi-square analyses conducted at baseline indicated. The MCI group received intervention over 2 years that focused on three domains (behavior problems, preacademic readiness skills, and child safety), delivered in both home and preschool or day care settings. Thus, this group received many of the early intervention components across all three tiers as described in previous chapters. Specifically, parent education consisted of twenty 2-hour sessions focused on behavior management, preacademics, and child safety (a longer term version of Tier 1 intervention described in Chapter 3 along with the academic and safety components described in Chapters 5 and 6, respectively). The Community Parent Education (COPE; C. E. Cunningham, 2006) curriculum was used, supplemented with sessions pertaining to ADHD information (e.g., characteristics, prevalence), functional assessment, injury prevention, and early literacy/numeracy skills. In addition to parent education, functional assessments and functional analyses were conducted in the children's homes. On the basis of the information gathered, individualized functional assessment-derived interventions were developed (as described for Tier 3 in Chapter 3). Parents were coached through implementation of the interventions. Finally, functional assessments were conducted in the preschool or day care and individualized interventions designed (as described for Tier 3 in Chapter 4). As were parents, preschool teachers and care providers were coached through accurate intervention implementation.

The PE group received only parent education over the course of 2 years. Thus, this group received a longer term version of Tier 1 home-based intervention described in Chapter 3. As with the MCI group, twenty 2-hour sessions were conducted. The Early Childhood Systematic Training for Effective Parenting (Dinkmeyer, McKay, Dinkmeyer, Dinkmeyer, & McKay, 1997) curriculum was used, with sessions pertaining to general child rearing (understanding child behavior, discipline, social–emotional development). This was supplemented with sessions pertaining to ADHD information (e.g., characteristics, prevalence), child health and nutrition, cognitive and language development, safety, parent self-care, and preparation for school.

Treatment outcomes were evaluated using many of the measures described in Chapter 1, including (a) standardized assessments in the form of questionnaires completed by parents and preschool and day care teachers, (b) preacademic skills assessments administered to children, and (c) direct observations. Analyses of 1- and 2-year outcomes were conducted using hierarchical linear modeling. Results indicated there were no significant group differences between the two treatment groups at 1 year after the onset of intervention (Kern et al., 2007). Importantly, statistically significant growth ($p < .01$) occurred for almost all of the dependent measures (16 of 18) examined at that time point. That is, negative trajectories were found for aggressive behavior, delinquent behavior, ADHD problems, oppositional defiant problems, and conduct problems, as measured by the Child Behavior Checklist (Achenbach, 1991a), the Teacher Rating Form (Achenbach, 1991b), and the Conners Rating Scales—Revised Long Form (Conners, 1997). In addition, statistically significant positive slopes were obtained for teacher- and parent-rated social skills (Social Skills Rating System—Parent Form and Teacher Form; Gresham & Elliott, 1990) and early literacy skills, including initial sound fluency, letter naming fluency, and phoneme segmentation fluency (Dynamic Indicators of Basic Early Literacy Skills (Kaminski & Good, 1996). The only areas in which significant slopes were not obtained were in the areas of delinquent behavior and school readiness (Bracken Basic Concepts Scale-Revised; Bracken, 1998).

Similar results were obtained for an expanded set of 46 dependent measures assessed every 6 months over 2 years. Specifically, statistically significant ($p < .05$) linear slope was found for 30 measures, all of which were in the expected direction (i.e., negative slope for parent and teacher behavior problem ratings as well as observations of noncompliant and off-task child behavior with positive slopes for parent and teacher ratings of social skills and direct assessment of academic skills). Significant quadratic slope (indicating a change in direction of slope) was found for 14 of the measures. Typically, these showed initial steep changes with slopes gradually tapering off over time.

Significant differences between the MCI and PE groups in linear or quadratic slope (or both) were found for nine measures, including ratings of parent stress and family coping, teacher ratings of oppositional behavior, and direct observations of off-task, noncompliance, and positive social engagement in preschool and home settings. Most of these differences in 2-year outcome favored the MCI group, including family coping, ratings of parent distress and problematic parent–child interactions, direct observations of classroom off-task behavior and positive behavior in parent–child interactions, and teacher ratings of oppositional behavior. Two years after the onset of treatment, the percentage of children meeting *DSM–IV* criteria for ADHD and ODD was reduced from 100% at baseline to 61.5% (ADHD) and from 76% to 46.2% (ODD). Further, following 2 years of treatment, only 8.3% of the sample would have met the initial inclusion criteria (i.e., *DSM–IV* criteria plus extreme parent and teacher behavior ratings) for entry into the study. None of the participants met criteria for CD after 2 years, and only 29.1% were receiving psychotropic medication. Although there were no statistically significant differences between groups with respect to diagnostic and medication outcomes, the direction of differences in most cases favored the MCI group. Also, the rates of diagnosis and impairment (see Figure 9.1) as well as percentage of children receiving psychotropic medication (see Figure 9.2) were less than that obtained by Lahey et al. (2004) with their untreated sample of young children with ADHD followed over a 2-year period.

These findings indicate that early intervention had a significant impact on home and preschool behavioral functioning and possibly on preacademic and home safety skills. In general, children in both groups improved significantly, in contrast to the more typical flatline or worsening of behavioral outcomes found in this population (e.g., see Lahey et al., 2004). Although there were few differences between the two early intervention groups, the MCI approach may be stronger for certain outcomes (e.g., noncompliance, off-task behavior, and reduction of medication use) in the second year of treatment, particularly in the preschool or elementary school setting. These outcomes suggest that certain subgroups experienced differential benefits from this more

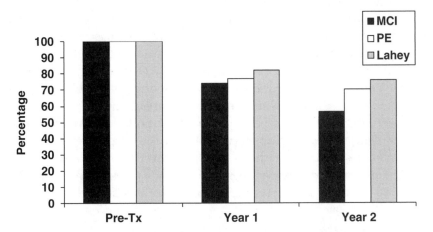

*Figure 9.1.* Percentage of children meeting *Diagnostic and Statistical Manual of Mental Disorders* (4th ed., text revision) criteria for attention-deficit/hyperactivity disorder plus significant impairment as a function of group and time. MCI = multicomponent intervention; PE = parent education; Lahey = participants in Lahey et al. (2004) longitudinal study; Tx = diagnosis.

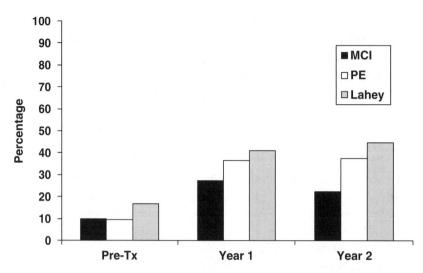

*Figure 9.2.* Percentage of participants receiving psychotropic medication. MCI = multicomponent intervention; PE = parent education; Lahey = participants in Lahey et al. (2004) longitudinal study; Tx = diagnosis.

intensive intervention. Further, parents in the MCI group rated treatment strategies as significantly more acceptable than parents in the PE group at the 6- and 12-month assessment phases. No significant group differences in treatment acceptability were found at 18 and 24 months. Overall treatment acceptability for both groups was in the moderate range. Teachers also reported MCI intervention strategies to be moderately acceptable and effective.

Individual response to treatment varied considerably within both groups. We calculated individual effect sizes for 6-month outcomes for each participant using parent and teacher ratings of oppositional behaviors (Conners T scores). Ratings of oppositional behavior were used because behaviors targeted for intervention were primarily noncompliance and aggression. Effect sizes were calculated using the following formula: (pretreatment rating – 6-month treatment rating) / Group standard deviation). A positive treatment response was identified for those participants who obtained an effect size of 0.5 standard deviation units or greater. In the PE group, 27% of the sample showed a positive response based on parent ratings, 42% based on teacher ratings, and 9.1% responded positively in both settings. Results were similar for the MCI group, with 27.5% showing a positive response based on parent ratings, 33.9% on teacher ratings, and 7.1% in both settings.

These intervention findings were notably promising for several reasons. They also raise critical questions for future research. First, significant improvements were seen for some children who received an intervention of relatively mild intensity, in the form of parent education. Given that sessions were conducted with groups of as many as 14 parents, this represents a cost-efficient form of prevention and intervention. At the same time, a subset of children did not respond to intervention, including some in the MCI group who received individualized assessment-based interventions in both home and school. Thus, it is imperative to further evaluate responsiveness to varying intensities of intervention. A second question that emerged from the findings was whether a less intensive parent education program would be equally effective in light of variable education session attendance among parents. Specifically, some children responded to a relatively low-intensity intervention and thus may not require twenty 2-hour sessions over an extended period of time. In fact, a three-tier early intervention model may be viable wherein children who exhibit a sufficient response to only parent and teacher education remain in that protocol, whereas children who are not responsive to parent and teacher education alone move to more intensive intervention strategies as described previously for Tiers 2 and 3. This tiered approach has the additional potential advantage of greater cost-effectiveness and feasibility given the limited resources for early intervention in the community.

### Predictors of Treatment Response

In an attempt to identify factors that could highlight children likely to respond to early intervention, an initial analysis of possible predictors of treatment response in the previously described data set examined the following pretreatment variables as predictors: age at study entry, IQ, parent stress, level of family support, ADHD symptom severity (parent reported), ADHD symptom severity (teacher reported), and total contact hours with consultant (as a proxy for treatment "dosage"). The degree to which these variables predicted 24-month outcome (i.e., intercept) and growth (i.e., slope) was examined for four criterion variables: Conners Oppositional $T$ Score (parent), Conners Oppositional $T$ Score (teacher), Woodcock–Johnson Test of Educational Achievement (WJ–III; Woodcock, McGrew, & Mather, 2001) calculation raw score, and WJ–III Letter–word identification raw score. Statistically significant ($p < .05$) predictors for parent ratings of oppositional behavior included parent stress (intercept), parental report of severity of ADHD symptoms (slope), and number of consultant contact hours (slope). The higher the level of parent stress at pretreatment, the higher the ratings of oppositional behavior at 24 months, highlighting the importance of family factors as discussed in Chapter 8. Children with more severe ADHD symptoms at pretreatment showed slower reduction in oppositional behavior across treatment. The more consultant contact hours, the steeper the decline in oppositional behavior, suggesting a treatment dosage effect for this variable. For teacher ratings of oppositional behavior, only teacher-rated pretreatment severity of ADHD symptoms was found to predict slope across 24 months. Specifically, children with more severe ADHD symptoms exhibited slower decline in oppositional behavior across treatment. Thus, children with more severe ADHD symptoms are going to be less likely to show immediate change and will most likely require more intensive Tiers 2 and 3 interventions.

Significant predictors of treatment effects for WJ–III letter–word identification included IQ (intercept), age at study entry (intercept and slope), and pretreatment teacher rating of ADHD symptom severity (intercept and slope). Children with higher cognitive ability and older children at study entry showed higher WJ–III scores at 24 months. Older children also exhibited steeper growth in letter–word identification across the 24-month period. Surprisingly, children with more severe ADHD symptoms showed higher WJ–III scores at 24 months and steeper growth. Predictors of treatment effects for WJ–III calculation included IQ (intercept), age at study entry (intercept and slope), parent-rated ADHD symptom severity (intercept), and teacher-rated ADHD symptom severity (intercept). Children with greater cognitive ability, lower ADHD symptom severity at home, and higher ADHD symptom severity at preschool obtained higher calculation scores at 24 months. Older children at study entry exhibited higher scores at 24 months and steeper growth of calculation skills. Thus, on the basis of this analysis of our current early intervention study, the following variables appear to be viable candidates as predictors of treatment response: age, IQ, ADHD symptom severity, parent stress, and number of consultant contact hours (i.e., a metric of treatment "dosage"). These variables may also help identify those children who are likely to require more intensive early intervention beyond Tier 1.


## MAJOR THEMES IN EARLY INTERVENTION FOR ADHD

### Early Assessment and Identification

Although research examining the effectiveness of intervention for young children with characteristics of ADHD is just emerging, available data suggest that it is highly effective both for reducing symptoms already present and preventing more serious problems from developing (e.g., Kern et al., 2007). Hence, assessment and identification of ADHD symptoms at the earliest age possible is critical. Recent research has indicated that symptoms of ADHD emerge and can be detected when children are very young (Egger, Kondo, & Angold, 2006; Spira & Fischel, 2005; Wolraich, 2006). For example, in a comprehensive evaluation of published research with children ages 2 to 5 years, Egger et al. (2006) found that the topography of symptoms seen in young children is consistent with symptoms described in the *DSM–IV–TR*. Further, Egger et al.'s research showed that early symptoms of ADHD can be reliably assessed, are associated with significant impairment, and occur outside of the normative range for preschool-age children. Finally, the ADHD-related characteristics seen in younger children mirror those of older children with respect to prevalence rates, subtypes, and gender differences, which further supports early emergence.

Despite the aforementioned work in this area, early identification remains tenuous, partly because young children, in general, are very active, and many have difficulties sustaining attention for longer than brief periods of time (Lahey et al., 1998). Further, only recently has the importance of early intervention been recognized, and, as we continue to realize the value of prevention, the process of identifying early ADHD symptoms will become more precise (Dunlap et al., 2006), as it is with other disorders (e.g., autism). Thus, at the current time, rather than focus on diagnosis, we recommend that practitioners become skilled at identifying early symptoms of ADHD (e.g., inattention, high levels of activity) and assessing the degree to which those behaviors exceed normative ranges and interfere with typical development and functioning. The best approach is a comprehensive and multimodal assessment that includes diagnostic interviews and behavior rating scales completed with both parents and preschool teachers, coupled with direct observations of child behavior, as described in Chapter 1. Intervention should then be delivered to those children with significant symptoms, and, when successful, diagnosis may be avoided.

## Potential Outcomes of Early Intervention

As we described in the Introduction to this book, early symptoms of ADHD include inattention (e.g., difficulty sustaining attention during play, failure to follow through after being given an instruction, appearing not to be listening, frequently losing toys) and hyperactivity or impulsivity (e.g., fidgety, excessive talking, high rates of motor movement, difficulty waiting). As a result of coercive parent–child interactions and impaired development, these behaviors frequently progress to more serious problems, such as aggression, defiance, poor peer relations, and failure to acquire early academic readiness skills (Campbell, Ewing, Breaux, & Szumowski, 1986; McGee, Partridge, Williams, & Silva, 1991). Depending on the severity of the problems, many children with early ADHD symptoms develop ODD and CD (e.g., Lahey & Loeber, 1997). Without early academic skills, later achievement in school is greatly compromised, and the achievement gap continues to widen (e.g., Kame'enui, 1993). Similar challenges continue as children age, resulting in chronic academic difficulties and social impairment continuing throughout life. Adolescent and adult difficulties include a high rate of school dropout, difficulties obtaining and maintaining employment, and comorbid psychiatric challenges, such as depression (e.g., Barkley, Murphy, & Fischer, 2008; McGee, Partridge, Williams, & Silva, 1991).

The goal of early intervention is to alter these typical social, behavioral, and academic trajectories. Research supports the premise that early symptoms can be significantly reduced, thus preventing more serious problems from developing (e.g., Kern et al., 2007). Further, research supports that early intervention can lead to continued reductions in behavior over time (see "Early Intervention for ADHD Project," as described previously). It is important to recognize that these changes in usual trajectories of problem behavior can be attributed to the alteration of environmental variables that contribute to and exacerbate problem behavior. That is, the etiology of ADHD involves an interaction between heritable and environmental factors (Nigg, 2006). Extensive evidence indicates that behavioral and academic interventions can alter environmental variables such that symptoms of ADHD are reduced and more serious problems are prevented (Sonuga-Barke, Daley, Thompson, Laver-Bradbury, & Weeks, 2001).

## Focus of Early Intervention

Research suggests that ADHD symptoms rarely occur in isolation (Barkley, 2006). The three primary challenges and risks that young children with ADHD symptoms experience are conduct problems, academic difficulties, and physical injuries. Not only are these core areas problematic at an early age, they also result in significant later problems and should be the focus of intervention efforts.

With respect to conduct problems, coercive exchanges between children and their parents or teachers can exacerbate problems (Patterson, Reid, & Dishion, 1992). Further, child behavior problems are associated with ineffective parenting practices as well as parent psychopathology and parent stress, which appears to represent a reciprocal relationship (Cummings & Davies, 1999). Thus, the focus on reducing child conduct problems improves children's social relationships and sets the stage for academic learning but also affects parenting practices and general parent well-being (Patterson et al., 1992).

Early academic skill deficits also are common among young children with ADHD symptoms. Deficits occur primarily in the areas of prereading, early math, and fine motor skills (DuPaul et al., 2001; Mariani & Barkley, 1997). There is a clear relationship between early academic skills and later academic achievement in that children with early academic skill deficits generally experience poor academic achievement throughout their school years (Kame'enui, 1993; McGill-Franzen, 1987). Thus, intervention in this area is critical for school and postschool success. Preacademic learning experiences can be incorporated into everyday activities and routines (Notari-Syverson, O'Connor, & Vadasy, 1998), adding little additional burden to parent responsibilities. Also, parents should be encouraged to seek preschools that offer structured preacademic experiences.

The third common challenge among preschool children with ADHD symptoms is accidental injuries and poisonings, most likely resulting from impulsive and overactive behavior (e.g., Szatmari, Offord, & Boyle, 1989). Injury prevention and safety promotion strategies are should be part of early intervention. Comprehensive programs such as The Injury Prevention Program (American Academy of Pediatrics, 1999a; http://www.aap.org/family/ tippmain.htm) offer materials to assess risk and strategies to identify and prevent common potential injuries.

Because problems in each of the areas of conduct, preacademic skills, and accidents are common, children's status and risk in each of these core areas should be assessed. As we described in Chapters 3 and 4, problems within each area should be prioritized. As more serious behavior problems are reduced, less problematic issues can then be addressed.

## Cross-Setting Intervention

In Chapter 1, we noted that one requirement to meet *DSM–IV–TR* criteria for ADHD is the presence of symptoms in two or more settings, such as home and preschool. In settings that lack structure and expectations, a typical child's behavior may resemble that of a child with ADHD. For example, in preschool settings without planned activities or expectations for behavioral deportment, children may become overly active (e.g., running about), fail to listen or follow instructions, use a loud volume tone, and engage in risky play behaviors (e.g., climbing, using materials inappropriately). These behaviors are symptomatic of a poorly managed setting rather than the disorder of ADHD, and intervention should focus on improving the setting by introducing structure and expectations.

Children who are truly ADHD symptomatic will exhibit impairment across multiple settings, and intervention is most beneficial when implemented in each setting. Cross-setting intervention provides the opportunity for consistent and pervasive behavioral expectations. That is, children have the opportunity to learn and practice age-appropriate expectations throughout all waking hours. Further, learning differs across settings, and children's later success requires access to setting-relevant instruction. For example, instruction at home usually focuses on skills such as self-help (e.g., dressing independently), whereas instruction in preschool centers should be more heavily focused on academic readiness (e.g., letter identification) and social skills (e.g., peer interactions). Intervention is needed across these settings to maximize children's comprehensive skill base.

In addition to reducing child behavior problems, home-based instruction may help reduce parent stress and other variables that interfere with effective family functioning (see Chapter 8). Further, preschool intervention is critical because children with ADHD symptoms are at high risk for suspension and expulsion (e.g., Lahey et al., 1998). Reducing problem behaviors will increase the likelihood that children stay in preschool, where they can learn critical social and preacademic skills.

We described intervention in home (Chapter 3) and preschool or day care settings (Chapter 4) because children spend most of their time in these two environments. At the same time, it is important for intervention to extend to other settings that are problematic, such as the homes of friends and family members and the community (e.g., grocery store). We embedded examples of such interventions in Chapter 3. In light of the fact that many families who have children with behavior problems avoid activities outside of the home (Lahey et al., 1998; Neely-Barnes & Dia, 2008), it is imperative that intervention address children's specific problems in all settings.

### Reduction in Medication Use

The PATS, a recent large-scale study (Kollins et al., 2006), was the first to comprehensively examine the use of stimulant medication (methylphenidate) in a large sample of preschool-age children with ADHD. Study findings indicated significant reductions in ADHD symptoms as well as possible adverse side effects, the most common being decreased appetite, difficulty sleeping, and weight loss. In addition, little is known about the long-term effects (i.e., longer than 1–2 months) of medication administration in this age group because of the absence of research. Further, children in the PATS showed considerable differences in their responsiveness to medications. In sum, the research to date indicates that medications are not universally effective and can result in significant side effects, and outcomes have been studied for limited time periods (see Chapter 7).

For the reasons listed previously, early behavioral intervention should be the initial course of action before even considering medication use (Kollins & Greenhill, 2006; Rappley et al., 2002). Specifically, young children with symptoms of ADHD should progress through Tiers 1, 2, and 3 interventions in the home and preschool setting (Chapters 3 and 4). In addition, evidence should support that the interventions are implemented with integrity, as designed. It is only when serious behavior problems persist following Tier 3 intervention that medications should be considered as a supplement to behavioral intervention. That is, although medication may reduce symptoms of ADHD (e.g., hyperactivity) in some children, it does not replace skill instruction. Instead, medication should be considered a supplement to behavioral intervention.

Overall, for many children, effective early intervention will delay or obviate the need for medication.

### Tiered Intervention

A tiered approach to intervention is one in which increasingly intensive intervention is provided only as needed. We described a three-tier approach, which is used in elementary schools throughout the United States. Tier 1, or *universal intervention*, is implemented with an entire population (e.g., classroom or program, all parents) and involves evidence-based strategies, such as teaching basic behavior management strategies to parents or establishing classwide or programwide expectations. Tier 2, or *secondary intervention*, is implemented only with those children who are not responsive to Tier 1. Tier 2 involves parent coaching in behavioral strategies or small-group instruction in schools. Finally, Tier 3, or *tertiary intervention*, is used with the small group of individuals who are not responsive to Tier 1 or Tier 2 interventions. At this tier, home and school interventions are assessment based and individualized.

This model of intervention is particularly effective and efficient for many reasons. First, Tier 1 is focused on teaching all children what is expected in preschool settings and teaching parents basic effective behavior management principles. Thus, all children receive intervention in the form of skill instruction. This is advantageous because it does not assume that children enter preschool understanding social and preacademic expectations (e.g., sharing, sitting, paying attention, following instructions), nor does it presume that parents are readily able to implement interventions for their children with chronic behavioral issues. Further, Tier 1 intervention is focused on preventing problem behavior, rather than merely responding after it occurs. As needed, children who do not respond to Tier 1 intervention systematically move to Tiers 2 and 3. Thus, the model is structured so that less intrusive and less costly approaches are implemented first, with interventions that require more time and effort implemented only for those children who do not respond to less intrusive efforts. This allows limited resources to be allocated in a cost-efficient manner.

## FUTURE DIRECTIONS

Although significant progress has been made in developing effective early intervention for young children with ADHD, important areas need to be addressed to enhance both research and, ultimately, clinical services with this population. First, treatment outcome studies (including clinical trials of medication) should focus on ameliorating functional impairments (e.g., academic and social performance deficits) in lieu of an exclusive focus on reducing ADHD symptoms. In some cases, improvement in ADHD symptoms leads to enhanced functioning in other areas; however, this outcome cannot be assumed. Thus, studies should directly target and assess children's functioning across academic, behavioral, and social realms.

Second, given that pharmacotherapy may have limitations (e.g., more frequent adverse side effects and lower parent acceptability) for treating ADHD in young children, early intervention studies should include *need for or delay to medication* as an outcome measure. Need for or delay to medication would be defined as the length of time between onset of early psychosocial intervention and the referral for or prescription of medication to treat ADHD. By including this outcome, studies could demonstrate whether effective psychosocial intervention in early childhood delays or obviates the need for psychotropic medication.

More detailed studies of behavioral and academic interventions need to be conducted with young children as has been done with elementary school–age children with ADHD. Although efficacy data support the general use of behavioral and academic interventions to treat ADHD and related impairments in early childhood, many important questions remain. For example, comparisons of several behavioral interventions (e.g., token reinforcement, response cost) could identify the optimal approach to address specific target behaviors in this population. Investigations could also help determine the best combinations of behavioral and academic interventions for specific subgroups of young children with ADHD (e.g., those with ADHD alone relative to children with ADHD and one or more associated disorders).

Intervention studies need to address specific risk variables that might affect treatment outcome. Our initial analyses of treatment predictors identified several important risk factors, including children's symptom severity and cognitive abilities, as well as the pretreatment level of parent stress. As an example of additional possible risk factors, parents who exhibit significant ADHD symptoms themselves or suffer from depression may have difficulties implementing structured behavioral strategies. Thus, a comprehensive treatment approach should include components that directly target risk variables or, at the very least, facilitate parents' receiving necessary treatment for their own difficulties. The identification of risk factors that may deleteriously affect early intervention or variables that may predict treatment response is critical to the design of comprehensive treatment programs.

In similar fashion, the efficacy of early intervention may be enhanced by a shift in focus from symptoms and outcomes to putative underlying causes (Sonuga-Barke & Halperin, 2010). To the extent that deficits in neuropsychological processes are demonstrated as mediators related to symptoms and impairment, early intervention that ameliorates these deficits could alter developmental trajectories such that children no longer have ADHD. Sonuga-Barke and Halperin (2010) provided a compelling rationale and description for early intervention that is individualized by targeting within-child variables that may underlie symptoms in different subgroups of young children at risk for ADHD. The Sonuga-Barke and Halperin model for early intervention is intriguing; however, extensive empirical work is necessary to demonstrate the veracity of the assumptions and components of this model.

Early intervention procedures may also differ on the basis of ADHD subtypes or differences in symptomatic trajectories over time. Sonuga-Barke, Auerbach, Campbell, Daley, and Thompson (2005) proposed different interventions for four variations of preschool ADHD. Specifically, some young children may exhibit subclinical levels of ADHD symptoms along with emerging oppositional defiant behavior. These children may respond best to parent education in behavior management along the lines of our proposed Tier 1 intervention. A second group of young children may exhibit the onset of significant ADHD symptoms as they approach school age and may respond best to interventions and strategies designed to address home-to-school transitions. A third group may only show ADHD symptoms during early childhood, which remit as the children mature. Again, this latter group may be helped best by providing parents with coping and behavior management strategies as in Tier 1. Finally, a fourth group of young children may develop ADHD symptoms early in life that are unremitting and chronic. Such children may require multiple tiers of intervention (i.e., more intensive psychosocial treatment) and possibly stimulant medication. These hypothetical linkages between subgroups and treatments are conceptually appealing but require empirical study.

Interventions that have been found effective in treating ADHD in older age groups could be adapted to be developmentally appropriate for use with young children. For example, self-regulation interventions (e.g., self-monitoring, self-evaluation) can improve ADHD-related behaviors and associated academic or social deficits in some elementary and middle school–age children with ADHD (for reviews, see DuPaul, Arbolino, & Booster, 2009; R. Reid, Trout, & Schartz, 2005). In similar fashion, treatment strategies that are effective for disorders closely related to ADHD (e.g., ODD, CD, learning disabilities) may be adapted for use with this population. By identifying potential application of interventions effective with other age groups or disabilities, early intervention approaches for ADHD can be expanded to be more comprehensive and potentially more effective in the long term.

Our early intervention for ADHD program emphasizes the use of a tiered approach in which children's response to intervention determines the content and intensity of treatment (see Chapter 2). Although our research, as well as studies conducted by other investigative teams, has supported a three-tiered early intervention protocol, additional work is needed to develop the best models for optimizing outcomes. For example, more information is needed to identify a clear, operational definition of *treatment response* that can be used to determine movement from tier to tier. The specific response or responses may vary across children based on individual need; however, a consistent method for operationalizing response should be developed to optimize the use of a three-tiered intervention program. Further, additional research is needed to identify optimal interventions at each tier, particularly Tiers 1 and 2. Little research has been conducted in preschool settings to identify effective classwide and programwide interventions, In addition, research is needed to support the particular types of Tier 2, small-group interventions that are most effective.

A final critical direction for development of effective early intervention is for research findings to be used in practice (i.e., in preschool classrooms and homes). Translational research studies should be conducted to identify feasible, cost-efficient methods to employ evidence-based strategies in real-world settings. We believe that a three-tiered approach to early intervention can help in this process by delivering more expensive, resource-intensive strategies only to those in greatest need. Nevertheless, research and dissemination efforts will be critical to determining the most feasible and effective ways to implement and promote tiered intervention, particularly in locations where services are most needed (e.g., urban, lower socioeconomic status communities).

## SUMMARY AND CONCLUSIONS

Assessment and intervention for young children with symptoms of ADHD have advanced considerably in recent years. Symptoms of ADHD can be detected early and reliably assessed. When intervention is delivered when behavior problems first emerge, more serious problems can be prevented. Recent research (e.g., Kern et al., 2007) has shown that intervention implemented during the preschool years can alter the trajectories of behavior problems that are common as children with ADHD age, such as the development of ODD and CD.

New models of intervention are effective and cost-efficient. That is, a tiered model of support ensures that all children receive instruction to prevent problem behavior. Increasingly intensive interventions are implemented only when children are nonresponsive to less intrusive intervention. When specific intervention strategies effective with young children with ADHD symptoms are embedded within this approach, symptoms can be greatly reduced and trajectories of problem behavior altered in a positive direction. This approach has proved highly effective, particularly for older children with problem behavior, and holds great promise for young children with ADHD symptoms.

Although emerging research in the early assessment and treatment of ADHD is promising, additional research is needed in several areas. In the area of intervention, a tiered model of support needs further study, particularly as it applies to young children with challenges such as ADHD. Research supporting its effectiveness with school-age children is rapidly emerging; however, research in preschools is limited. Additional study is needed to ensure that intervention at each tier is optimally designed to address the particular symptoms that young children with or at risk for ADHD exhibit. Also, specific interventions and combinations of interventions proven effective with older children with ADHD will benefit from further evaluation with young children. Intervention examination should also consider whether intervention is effective with each subtype of ADHD. Finally, risk variables need to be further researched, particularly to determine whether they can be eliminated or ameliorated.

Targeting and effectiveness of intervention warrant further study. It may be that targeting underlying causes of ADHD, such as neuropsychological sources, will be a parsimonious approach. Much research is needed, however, to determine the potential of this avenue. Meanwhile, the target of intervention must be broadened to include academic and social areas, beyond the current focus that primarily focuses on reducing symptoms of ADHD (e.g., overactivity, inattention). Finally, intervention effectiveness should be comprehensively measured, considering a broad variety of outcomes (e.g., how often the need for medication can be obviated) and long-term success (e.g., graduation rate, adult functioning).

Early intervention for ADHD is still in the formative stages. Although the research base is rapidly growing, there is a great deal left to learn. Nonetheless, research has clearly demonstrated that early intervention can reduce the more serious problems that generally follow a diagnosis of ADHD. Therefore, children with ADHD and their families will benefit greatly as the translation of current research into practice leads to increasingly effective and efficient interventions.

# REFERENCES

Abikoff, H., Gittelman-Klein, R., & Klein, D. F. (1977). Validation of a classroom observation code for hyperactive children. *Journal of Consulting and Clinical Psychology, 45,* 772–783. doi:10.1037/0022-006X.45.5.772

Abikoff, H. B., Vitiello, B., Riddle, M. A., Cunningham, C., Greenhill, L. L., Swanson, J. M., . . . & Wigal, T. (2007). Methylphenidate effects on functional outcomes in the Preschoolers with Attention-Deficit/Hyperactivity Disorder Treatment Study (PATS). *Journal of Child and Adolescent Psychopharmacology, 17,* 581–592. doi:10.1089/cap.2007.0068

Achenbach, T. M. (1991a). *Manual for the Child Behavior Checklist/4-18 and 1991 Profile.* Burlington: University of Vermont, Department of Psychiatry.

Achenbach, T. M. (1991b). *Manual for the Teacher's Report Form and 1991 Profile.* Burlington: University of Vermont, Department of Psychiatry.

Achenbach, T. M., & Rescorla, L. A. (2000). *Manual for the ASEBA preschool forms and profiles.* Burlington: Research Center for Children, Youth, & Families, University of Vermont.

Alpert, C. L., & Kaiser, A. P. (1992). Training parents as milieu language teachers. *Journal of Early Intervention, 16,* 31–52.

American Academy of Pediatrics. (1999a). *TIPP: The Injury Prevention Program.* Elk Grove, IL: Author.

American Academy of Pediatrics. (1999b). *TIPP safety surveys.* Elk Grove, IL: Author.

American Psychiatric Association. (2000). *Diagnostic and statistical manual of mental disorders* (4th ed., text revision). Washington, DC: Author.

Anastopoulos, A. D., Guevremont, D. C., Shelton, T. L., & DuPaul, G. J. (1992). Parenting stress among families of children with attention deficit hyperactivity disorder. *Journal of Abnormal Child Psychology, 20,* 503–520. doi:10.1007/BF00916812

Anastopoulos, A. D., & Shelton, T. L. (2001). *Assessing attention-deficit/hyperactivity disorder.* New York, NY: Kluwer Academic/Plenum.

Anderson, C. A., & Hammen, C. L. (1993). Psychosocial outcomes of children of unipolar depressed, bipolar, medically ill, and normal women: A longitudinal study. *Journal of Consulting and Clinical Psychology, 61,* 448–454. doi:10.1037/0022-006X.61.3.448

Anderson, C. A., Hinshaw, S. P., & Simmel, C. (1994). Mother–child interactions in ADHD and comparison boys: Relationships with overt and covert externalizing behavior. *Journal of Abnormal Child Psychology, 22,* 247–265. doi:10.1007/BF02167903

Arcia, E., Reyes-Blanes, M., & Vazquez-Montilla, E. (2000). Constructions and reconstructions: Latino parent's values for children. *Journal of Child and Family Studies, 9,* 333–350. doi:10.1023/A:1026444507343

Baker, B. L., Blacher, J., & Olsson, M. B. (2005). Preschool children with and without developmental delay: Behavior problems, parents' optimism and well-being. *Journal of Intellectual Disability Research, 49*, 575–590. doi:10.1111/j.1365-2788.2005.00691.x

Baker-Ericzén, M. J., Brookman-Frazee, L., & Stahmer, A. (2005). Stress levels and adaptability in parents of toddlers with and without autism spectrum disorders. *Research and Practice for Persons With Severe Disabilities, 30*, 194–204. doi:10.2511/rpsd.30.4.194

Bambara, L. M., & Kern, L. (2005). *Individualized supports for students with problem behaviors.* New York, NY: Guilford Press.

Barkley, R. A. (1988). The effects of methylphenidate on the interactions of preschool ADHD children with their mothers. *Journal of the American Academy of Child and Adolescent Psychiatry, 27*, 336–341. doi:10.1097/00004583-198805000-00012

Barkley, R. A. (1997). Behavioral inhibition, sustained attention, and executive functions: Constructing a unifying theory of ADHD. *Psychological Bulletin, 121*, 65–94. doi:10.1037/0033-2909.121.1.65

Barkley, R. A. (2001). Accidents and ADHD. *The Economics of Neuroscience, 3*, 64–68.

Barkley, R. A. (Ed.). (2006). *Attention deficit hyperactivity disorder: A handbook for diagnosis and treatment* (3rd ed.). New York, NY: Guilford Press.

Barkley, R. A., & Murphy, K. R. (2006). *Attention-deficit hyperactivity disorder: A clinical workbook* (3rd ed.). New York, NY: Guilford Press.

Barkley, R. A., Murphy, K. R., & Fischer, M. (2008). *ADHD in adults: What the science says.* New York, NY: Guilford Press.

Barkley, R. A., Shelton, T. L., Crosswait, C. C., Morehouse, M., Fletcher, K., Barrett, S., . . . & Metevia, L. (2000). Multi-method psycho-educational intervention for preschool children with disruptive behavior: Preliminary results at post-treatment. *Journal of Child Psychology and Psychiatry, and Allied Disciplines, 41*, 319–332. doi:10.1111/1469-7610.00616

Beck, I., & Juel, C. (1999). The role of decoding in learning to read: Consortium on Reading Excellence (Eds.), *Reading research anthology: The why of reading instruction* (pp. 78–87). Novato, CA: Arena Press.

Biemiller, A. (2001). Teaching vocabulary: Early, direct, and sequential. *American Educator, 25*, 24–28, 47.

Bijur, P., Golding, J., Haslum, M., & Kurzon, M. (1988). Behavioral predictors of injury in school-age children. *American Journal of Diseases of Children, 142*, 1307–1312.

Blumberg, S., Olson, L., Frankel, M., Osborn, L., Srinath, K., & Giambo, P. (2005). *Design and operation of the National Survey of Children's Health, 2003* (Vital and Health Statistics Reports, Series 1, No. 43). Washington, DC: National Center for Health Statistics.

Boyajian, A. E., DuPaul, G. J., Wartel Handler, M., Eckert, T. L., & McGoey, K. E. (2001). The use of classroom-based brief functional analyses with preschoolers at-risk for attention deficit hyperactivity disorder. *School Psychology Review, 30,* 278–293.

Bracken, B. A. (1998). *Examiner's manual for the Bracken Basic Concept Scale—Revised.* San Antonio, TX: The Psychological Corporation, Harcourt Brace.

Bredekamp, S. E., & Copple, C. E. (1996). *Developmentally appropriate practice in early childhood programs.* Washington, DC: National Association for the Education of Young Children.

Breslin, F. C., Sobell, M. B., Sobell, L. C., Cunningham, J. A., Sdao-Jarvie, K., & Borsoi, D. (1998). Problem drinkers: Evaluation of a stepped-care approach. *Journal of Substance Abuse, 10,* 217–232. doi:10.1016/S0899-3289(99)00008-5

Brookman-Frazee, L. (2004). Using parent/clinician partnerships in parent education programs for children with autism. *Journal of Positive Behavior Interventions, 6,* 195–213. doi:10.1177/10983007040060040201

Brookman-Frazee, L., & Koegel, R. L. (2010). Using parent/clinician partnerships in parent education programs for children with autism. *Journal of Positive Behavior Interventions, 12,* 23–32.

Brown, R. T., Antonuccio, D. O., DuPaul, G. J., Fristad, M. A., King, C. A., Leslie, L. K., . . . & Vitiello, B. (2007). *Childhood mental health disorders: Evidence base and contextual factors for psychosocial, psychopharmacological, and combined interventions.* Washington, DC: American Psychological Association.

Bruder, M. B. (2000). Family-centered early intervention: Clarifying our values for the new millennium. *Topics in Early Childhood Special Education, 20,* 105–115. doi:10.1177/027112140002000206

Buhrmester, D., Camparo, L., Christensen, A., Gonzales, L. S., & Hinshaw, S. P. (1992). Mothers and fathers interacting in dyads and triads with normal and hyperactive sons. *Developmental Psychology, 28,* 500–509. doi:10.1037/0012-1649.28.3.500

Burge, D., & Hammen, C. (1991). Maternal communication: Predictors of outcome at follow-up in a sample of children at high and low risk for depression. *Journal of Abnormal Psychology, 100,* 174–180. doi:10.1037/0021-843X.100.2.174

Byrne, J. M., Bawden, H. N., Beattie, T., & DeWolfe, N. A. (2003). Risk for injury in preschoolers: Relationship to attention deficit hyperactivity disorder. *Child Neuropsychology, 9,* 142–151.

Caldwell, B. M., & Bradley, R. H. (2001). *HOME inventory administration manual* (3rd ed.). Little Rock: University of Arkansas.

The California Child Care Health Program. (1998). *Health and safety in the child care setting: Prevention of injuries.* Berkeley, CA: Author.

The California Child Care Health Program. (2007). *Health and safety in the child care setting: Prevention of injuries, Module 2* (2nd ed.). Berkeley CA: Author.

Campbell, S. B. (1995). Behavior problems in preschool children: A review of recent research. *Journal of Child Psychology and Psychiatry, and Allied Disciplines, 36,* 113–149. doi:10.1111/j.1469-7610.1995.tb01657.x

Campbell, S. B. (2002). *Behavior problems in preschool children: Clinical and developmental issues* (2nd ed.). New York, NY: Guilford Press.

Campbell, S. B., Endman, M., & Bernfield, G. (1977). A three-year follow-up of hyperactive preschoolers into elementary school. *Journal of Child Psychology and Psychiatry, and Allied Disciplines, 18,* 239–249. doi:10.1111/j.1469-7610.1977.tb00436.x

Campbell, S. B., & Ewing, L. J. (1990). Follow-up of hard to manage preschoolers: Adjustment at age 9 and predictors of continuing symptoms. *Journal of Child Psychology and Psychiatry, and Allied Disciplines, 31,* 871–889. doi:10.1111/j.1469-7610.1990.tb00831.x

Campbell, S. B., Ewing, L. J., Breaux, A. M., & Szumowski, E. K. (1986). Parent-referred problem three-year-olds: Follow-up at school entry. *Journal of Child Psychology and Psychiatry, and Allied Disciplines, 27,* 473–488. doi:10.1111/j.1469-7610.1986.tb00635.x

Campbell, S. B., Schleifer, M., & Weiss, G. (1978). Continuities in maternal reports and child behaviors over time in hyperactive and comparison groups. *Journal of Abnormal Child Psychology, 6,* 33–45. doi:10.1007/BF00915780

Castle, L., Aubert, R. E., Verbrugge, R. R., Khalid, M., & Epstein, R. S. (2007). Trends in medication treatment for ADHD. *Journal of Attention Disorders, 10,* 335–342. doi:10.1177/1087054707299597

Centers for Disease Control and Prevention. (2005, September 2). Mental health in the United States: Prevalence of diagnosis and medication treatment for attention-deficit/hyperactivity disorder—United States, 2003. *Morbidity and Mortality Weekly Report.* Retrieved from http://www.cdc.gov/mmwr/preview/mmwrhtml/mm5434a2.htm

Chan, S. (1990). Early intervention with culturally diverse families of infants and toddlers with disabilities. *Infants and Young Children, 3,* 78–87. doi:10.1097/00001163-199010000-00010

Chandler, L. K. (1992). Generalization and maintenance of preschool children's social skills: A critical review and analysis. *Journal of Applied Behavior Analysis, 25,* 415–428. doi:10.1901/jaba.1992.25-415

Chard, D. J., Harn, B. A., Sugai, G., Horner, R. H., Simmons, D. C., & Kame'enui, E. J. (2008). Core features of multi-tiered systems of reading and behavioral support. In C. R. Greenwood, T. R. Kratochwill, & M. Clemens (Eds.), *Schoolwide prevention models: Lessons learned in elementary schools* (pp. 31–60). New York, NY: Guilford Press.

Chen, D., Downing, J. E., & Peckham-Hardin, K. D. (2002). Working with families of diverse cultural and linguistic backgrounds. In J. M. Lucyshyn, G. Dunlap, & R. W. Albin (Eds.), *Families and positive behavior support* (pp. 133–154). Baltimore, MD: Brookes.

Chronis, A. M., Lahey, B. B., Pelham, W. E., Williams, S. H., Baumann, B. L., Kipp, H., . . . & Rathouz, P. J. (2007). Maternal depression and early positive parenting predict future conduct problems in young children with attention-deficit/ hyperactivity disorder. *Developmental Psychology, 43,* 70–82. doi:10.1037/0012-1649.43.1.70

Codding, R. S., Feinberg, A. B., Dunn, E. K., & Pace, G. M. (2005). Effects of immediate performance feedback on implementation of behavior support plans. *Journal of Applied Behavior Analysis, 38,* 205–219. doi:10.1901/jaba.2005.98-04

Collins, L. M., Murphy, S. A., & Bierman, K. L. (2004). A conceptual framework for adaptive preventive interventions. *Prevention Science, 5,* 185–196. doi:10.1023/B:PREV.0000037641.26017.00

Commission on Chronic Illness. (1957). *Chronic illness in the United States.* Cambridge, MA: Harvard University Press.

Conners, C. K. (1997). *Conners Rating Scales—revised technical manual.* North Tonawanda, NY: Multi-Health Systems.

Conners, C. K. (2001). *Conners Kiddie Continuous Performance Test.* Toronto, Ontario, Canada: Multi-Health Systems.

Conners, C. K. (2008). *Conners Comprehensive Behavior Rating Scale.* Toronto, Ontario, Canada: Multi-Health Systems.

Connor, D. F. (2006a). Other medications. In R. A. Barkley (Ed.), *Attention-deficit/hyperactivity disorder: A handbook for diagnosis and treatment* (3rd ed., pp. 658–677). New York, NY: Guilford Press.

Connor, D. F. (2006b). Stimulants. In R. A. Barkley (Ed.), *Attention-deficit/hyperactivity disorder: A handbook for diagnosis and treatment* (3rd ed., pp. 608–647). New York, NY: Guilford Press.

Correa, V. I. (1987). Working with Hispanic parents of visually impaired children: Cultural implications. *Journal of Visual Impairment & Blindness, 81,* 260–264.

Cotter, R. B., Burke, J. D., Loeber, R., & Navratil, J. L. (2002). Innovative retention methods in longitudinal research: A case study of the developmental trends study. *Journal of Child and Family Studies, 11,* 485–498.

Craig-Unkefer, L. A., & Kaiser, A. P. (2002). Improving the social communication skills of at-risk preschool children in a play context. *Topics in Early Childhood Special Education, 22,* 3–13. doi:10.1177/027112140202200101

Cummings, E. M., & Davies, P. T. (1999). Depressed parents and family functioning: Interpersonal effects and children's functioning and development. In T. Joiner & J. C. Coyne (Eds.), *The interactional nature of depression* (pp. 299–327). Washington, DC: American Psychological Association. doi:10.1037/10311-011

Cunningham, A. E., & Stanovich, K. E. (1998). What reading does for the mind. *American Educator, 22*(1–2), 8–15.

Cunningham, C. E. (2006). COPE: Large-group, community-based, family-centered parent training. In R. A. Barkley (Ed.), *Attention-deficit/hyperactivity disorder: A handbook for diagnosis and treatment* (3rd ed., pp. 480–498). New York, NY: Guilford Press.

Cunningham, C. E., & Barkley, R. A. (1979). The interactions of hyperactive and normal children with their mothers during free play and structured tasks. *Child Development, 50*, 217–224. doi:10.2307/1129059

Cunningham, C. E., Bremner, R. B., & Boyle, M. (1995). Large group community-based parenting programs for families of preschoolers at risk for disruptive behaviour disorders: Utilization, cost effectiveness, and outcome. *Journal of Child Psychology and Psychiatry, and Allied Disciplines, 36*, 1141–1159. doi:10.1111/j.1469-7610.1995.tb01362.x

Cunningham, C. E., Bremner, R., & Secord, M. (1998). *Community parent education program.* Hamilton, Ontario, Canada: Hamilton Health Sciences Corp.

Danforth, J. S., Barkley, R. A., & Stokes, T. F. (1991). Observations of parent–child interactions with hyperactive children: Research and clinical implications. *Clinical Psychology Review, 11*, 703–727. doi:10.1016/0272-7358(91)90127-G

Davidson, L. L., Hughes, S. J., & O'Connor, P. A. (1988). Preschool behavior problems and subsequent risk of injury. *Pediatrics, 82*, 644–651.

DeWolfe, N. A., Byrne, J. M., & Bawden, H. N. (1999). Early assessment of attention. *Clinical Neuropsychologist, 13*, 458–473.

DeWolfe, N. A., Byrne, J. M., & Bawden, H. N. (2000). Preschool inattention and impulsivity-hyperactivity: Development of a clinic-based assessment protocol. *Journal of Attention Disorders, 4*, 80–90. doi:10.1177/108705470000400202

Dinkmeyer, D., McKay, G. D., Dinkmeyer, J. S., Dinkmeyer, D., & McKay, J. L. (1997). *Early childhood systematic training for effective parenting (STEP).* Circle Pines, MN: American Guidance Services.

DiPerna, J. C., & Elliott, S. N. (2000). *Academic Competence Evaluation Scales.* San Antonio, TX: The Psychological Corporation.

DiScala, C., Lescohier, I., Barthel, M., & Li, G. (1998). Injuries to children with Attention deficit hyperactivity disorder. *Pediatrics, 102*, 1415–1421.

Dishion, T. J., French, D. C., & Patterson, G. R. (1996). The development and ecology of antisocial behavior. In D. Cicchetti & D. J. Cohen (Eds.), *Developmental psychopathology, Vol. 2. Risk, disorder, and adaptation* (pp. 421–471). New York, NY: Wiley.

Dishion, T. J., Patterson, G. R., & Kavanagh, K. A. (1992). An experimental test of the coercion model: Linking theory, measurement, and intervention. In J. McCord & R. E. Tremblay (Eds.), *Preventing antisocial behavior: Interventions from birth through adolescence* (pp. 253–282). New York, NY: Guilford Press.

Downey, G., & Coyne, J. C. (1990). Children of depressed parents: An integrative review. *Psychological Bulletin, 108*, 50–76. doi:10.1037/0033-2909.108.1.50

Drouin, M. A. (2009). Parent involvement in literacy intervention: A longitudinal study of effects on preschoolers' emergent literacy skills and home literacy environment. *Early Childhood Services: An Interdisciplinary Journal of Effectiveness, 3*, 1–18.

Dunlap, G., Harrower, J., & Fox, L. (2005). Understanding the environmental determinants of problem behavior. In L. M. Bambara & L. Kern (Eds.), *Individualized *supports for students with problem behaviors* (pp. 25–46). New York, NY: Guilford Press.

Dunlap, G., Strain, P. S., Fox, L., Carta, J. J., Conroy, M., Smith, B., . . . & Sowell, C. (2006). Prevention and intervention with young children's challenging behavior: perspectives regarding current knowledge. *Behavioral Disorders, 32,* 29–45.

Dunn, L., Beach, S. A., & Kontos, S. (2000). Supporting literacy in early childhood programs: A challenge for the future. In K. A. Roskos & J. F. Christie (Eds.), *Play and literacy in early childhood: Research from multiple perspectives* (pp. 91–105). Mahwah, NJ: Erlbaum.

Dunst, C. J., & Paget, K. (1991). Parent–professional partnerships and family empowerment. In M. J. Fine (Ed.), *Collaboration with parents of exceptional children* (pp. 25–44). Brandon, VT: Clinical Psychology.

DuPaul, G. J., Arbolino, L. A., & Booster, G. D. (2009). Cognitive–behavioral interventions for attention-deficit/hyperactivity disorder. In M. J. Mayer, R. Van Acker, J. E. Lochman, & F. M. Gresham (Eds.), *Cognitive–behavioral interventions for emotional and behavioral disorders: School-based practice* (pp. 295–327). New York, NY: Guilford Press.

DuPaul, G. J., Kern, L., Thomas, L. B., Caskie, G., & Rutherford, L. E. (2009, February). *Early intervention for young children with ADHD: 24-month outcomes.* Paper presented at the annual conference of the National Association of School Psychologists, Boston MA.

DuPaul, G. J., McGoey, K. E., Eckert, T. L., & VanBrakle, J. (2001). Preschool children with attention-deficit/hyperactivity disorder: Impairments in behavioral, social, and school functioning. *Journal of the American Academy of Child and Adolescent Psychiatry, 40,* 508–515. doi:10.1097/00004583-200105000-00009

DuPaul, G. J., Power, T. J., Anastopoulos, A. D., & Reid, R. (1998). *AD/HD Rating Scale—IV: Checklist, norms, and clinical interpretation.* New York, NY: Guilford Press.

DuPaul, G. J., & Stoner, G. (2003). *ADHD in the schools: Assessment and intervention strategies* (2nd ed.). New York, NY: Guilford Press.

Dyson, L. L. (1997). Fathers and mothers of school-age children with developmental disabilities: Parental stress, family functioning, and social support. *American Journal on Mental Retardation, 102,* 267–279. doi:10.1352/0895-8017(1997)102<0267:FAMOSC>2.0.CO;2

Egger, H. L., Kondo, D., & Angold, A. (2006). The epidemiology and diagnostic issues in preschool attention-deficit/hyperactivity disorder: A review. *Infants and Young Children, 19,* 109–122. doi:10.1097/00001163-200604000-00004

Elgar, F. J., McGrath, P. J., & Waschbusch, D. A. (2004). Mutual influences on maternal depression and child adjustment problems. *Clinical Psychology Review, 24,* 441–459. doi:10.1016/j.cpr.2004.02.002

Elliot, J., Prior, M., Merrigan, C., & Ballinger, K. (2002). Evaluation of a community intervention programme for preschool behavior problems. *Journal of Paediatrics and Child Health, 38,* 41–50.

Elliott, C. D. (1990). *The Differential Ability Scales*. San Antonio, TX: The Psychological Corporation.

Erchul, W. P. & Martens, B. K. (2010). School consultation: Conceptual and empirical bases for practice. In M. C. Roberts (Ed.), *Issues in child clinical psychology*. New York, NY: Springer.

Fabiano, G. A., Pelham, W. E., Jr., Gnagy, E. M., Burrows-MacLean, L., Coles, E. K., Chacko, A., . . . & Hoffman, M. T. (2007). The single and combined effects of multiple intensities of behavior modification and methylphenidate for children with attention deficit hyperactivity disorder in a classroom setting. *School Psychology Review, 36,* 195–216.

Fabiano, G. A., Pelham, W. E., Jr., Waschbusch, D. A., Gnagy, E. M., Lahey, B. B., Chronis, A. M., . . . & Burrows-MacLean, L. (2006). A practical measure of impairment: Psychometric properties of the Impairment Rating Scale in samples of children with attention deficit hyperactivity disorder and two school-based samples. *Journal of Clinical Child and Adolescent Psychology, 35,* 369–385. doi:10.1207/s15374424jccp3503_3

Faraone, S. V., Biederman, J., Jetton, J. G., & Tsuang, M. T. (1997). Attention deficit disorder and conduct disorder: Longitudinal evidence for a familial subtype. *Psychological Medicine, 27,* 291–300. doi:10.1017/S0033291796004515

Faraone, S. V., Perlis, R. H., Doyle, A. E., Smoller, J. W., Goralnick, J. J., Holmgren, M. A., & Sklar, P. (2005). Molecular genetics of attention-deficit/hyperactivity disorder. *Biological Psychiatry, 57,* 1313–1323. doi:10.1016/j.biopsych.2004.11.024

Feil, E. G., Walker, H. M., & Severson, H. H. (1995). The Early Screening Project for young children with behavior problems. *Journal of Emotional and Behavioral Disorders, 3,* 194–202.

Ferriero, E., & Teberosky, A. (1982). *Literacy before schooling*. Portsmouth, NH: Heinemann Educational Books.

Ferster, C. B., & Skinner, B. F. (1957). *Schedules of reinforcement*. Acton, MA: Copley. doi:10.1037/10627-000

Fischer, M. (1990). Parenting stress and the child with attention deficit hyperactivity disorder. *Journal of Clinical Child Psychology, 19,* 337–346. doi:10.1207/s15374424jccp1904_5

Fleming, J., & Monda-Amaya, L. E. (2001). Process variables critical for team effectiveness. *Remedial and Special Education, 22,* 158–171. doi:10.1177/074193250102200304

Floyd, R. G., Hojnoski, R. L., & Key, J. M. (2006). Preliminary evidence of technical adequacy of the Preschool Numeracy Indicators. *School Psychology Review, 35,* 627–644.

Foorman, B. R., & Torgesen, J. (2001). Critical elements of classroom and small-group instruction promote reading success in all children. *Learning Disabilities Research & Practice, 16,* 203–212.

Fox, L., Dunlap, G., Hemmeter, M. L., Joseph, G. E., & Strain, P. S. (2003). The teaching pyramid: A model for promoting social competence and preventing challenging behavior in young children. *Young Children, 3,* 48–52.

Fox, L., Jack, S., & Broyles, L. (2005). *Program-wide positive behavior support: Supporting young children's social–emotional development and addressing challenging behavior.* Tampa: Louis de la Parte Florida Mental Health Institute, University of South Florida.

Frazier, T. W., Youngstrom, E. A., Glutting, J. J., & Watkins, M. W. (2007). ADHD and achievement: Meta-analysis of the child, adolescent, and adult literatures and a concomitant study with college students. *Journal of Learning Disabilities, 40,* 49–65. doi:10.1177/00222194070400010401

Fuchs, D., & Fuchs, L. S. (2006). Introduction to response to intervention: What, why, and how valid is it? *Reading Research Quarterly, 41,* 93–99.

Gadow, K. D. (1986). *Children on medication: Vol. 1. Hyperactivity, learning disabilities, and mental retardation.* San Diego, CA: College-Hill Press.

Gadow, K. D., & Sprafkin, J. (1997). *Early Childhood Inventory—4: Norms manual.* Stony Brook, NY: Checkmate Plus.

Gallagher, P. A., Rhodes, C. A., & Darling, S. M. (2004). Parents as professionals in early intervention: A parent educator model. *Topics in Early Childhood Special Education, 24,* 5–13. doi:10.1177/02711214040240010101

Gallimore, R., Weisner, T. S., Kaufman, S. Z., & Bernheimer, L. P. (1989). The social construction of ecocultural niches: Family accommodation of developmentally delayed children. *American Journal on Mental Retardation, 94,* 216–230.

Garzon, D. L., Huang, H., & Todd, R. D. (2008). Do attention deficit/hyperactivity disorder and oppositional defiant disorder influence preschool unintentional injury risk? *Archives of Psychiatric Nursing, 22,* 288–296. doi:10.1016/j.apnu.2007.12.006

Gersten, R., & Chard, D. (1999). Number sense: Rethinking arithmetic instruction for students with mathematical disabilities. *The Journal of Special Education, 33,* 18–28. doi:10.1177/002246699903300102

Gersten, R., & Jordan, N. C. (2005). Early screening and intervention in mathematics difficulties: The need for action: Introduction to special series. *Journal of Learning Disabilities, 38,* 291–292.

Gersten, R., Jordan, N. C., & Flojo, J. R. (2005). Early identification and interventions for students with mathematics difficulties. *Journal of Learning Disabilities, 38,* 293–304. doi:10.1177/00222194050380040301

Ghuman, J. K., Arnold, L. E., & Anthony, B. J. (2008). Psychopharmacological and other treatments in preschool children with attention-deficit/hyperactivity disorder: Current evidence and practice. *Journal of Child and Adolescent Psychopharmacology, 18,* 413–447. doi:10.1089/cap.2008.022

Ghuman, J. K., Riddle, M. A., Vitiello, B., Greenhill, L. L., Chuang, S. Z., Wigal, S. B., . . . & Skorbala, A. M. (2007). Comorbidity moderates response to methylphenidate in the Preschoolers With Attention-Deficit/Hyperactivity Disorder Treatment Study (PATS). *Journal of Child and Adolescent Psychopharmacology, 17*, 563–580. doi:10.1089/cap.2007.0071

Gilliam, J. E. (1995). *Gilliam Autism Rating Scale*. Austin, TX: Pro-Ed.

Gilliam, W. S. (2005). *Prekindergarteners left behind: Expulsion rates in state prekindergarten classrooms*. New Haven, CT: Yale University Child Study Center. Retrieved from http://www.plan4preschool.org/documents/pk-expulsion.pdf

Gimpel, G. A., & Kuhn, B. R. (2000). Maternal report of attention deficit hyperactivity disorder symptoms in preschool children. *Child: Care, Health and Development, 26*, 163–176.

Gleason, M. M., Egger, H. L., Emslie, G. J., Greenhill, L. L., Kowatch, R. A., Lieberman, A. F., . . . & Zeanah, C. H. (2007). Psychopharmacological treatment for very young children: Contexts and guidelines. *Journal of the American Academy of Child and Adolescent Psychiatry, 46*, 1532–1572. doi:10.1097/chi.0b013e3181570d9e

Glover, T. A., & Vaughn, S. (2010). *The promise of response to intervention: Evaluating current science and practice*. New York, NY: Guilford Press.

Good, R. H., Simmons, C., & Smith, S. B. (1998). Effective academic intervention in the United States: Evaluating and enhancing the acquisition of early reading skills. *Educational and Child Psychology, 15*, 56–70.

Gordon, M. (1996). *Administrative manual for the Gordon Diagnostic System*. DeWitt, NY: Author.

Gordon, R. S. (1983). An operational classification of disease prevention. *Public Health Reports, 98*, 107–109.

Greenhill, L., Kollins, S., Abikoff, H., McCracken, J., Riddle, M., Swanson, J., . . . , & Cooper, T. (2006). Efficacy and safety of immediate-release methylphenidate treatment for preschoolers with ADHD. *Journal of the American Academy of Child and Adolescent Psychiatry, 45*, 1284–1293. doi:10.1097/01.chi.0000235077.32661.61

Greenhill, L. L., Posner, K., Vaughan, B. S., & Kratochvil, C. J. (2008). Attention deficit hyperactivity disorder in preschool children. *Child and Adolescent Psychiatric Clinics of North America, 17*, 347–366.

Gresham, F. M., & Elliott, S. N. (1990). *Social Skills Rating System manual*. Circle Pines, MN: American Guidance Service.

Gresham, F. M., & Elliott, S. N. (2008). *Social Skills Improvement System*. Minneapolis, MN: Pearson Assessments.

Griffin, S. (2004). Building number sense with number worlds: A mathematics program for young children. *Early Childhood Research Quarterly, 19*, 173–180.

Griffin, S. (2007). Early intervention for children at risk of developing mathematical learning difficulties. In D. B. Berch & M. M. M. Mazzocco (Eds.), *Why is math* so hard for some children? The nature and origins of mathematical learning difficulties and disabilities (pp. 373–395). Baltimore, MD: Brookes.

Groce, N. E., & Zola, I. K. (1993). Multiculturalism, chronic illness, and disability. Pediatrics, 91, 1048–1055.

Hailemariam, A., Bradley-Johnson, S., & Johnson, C. M. (2002). Pediatricians' preferences for ADHD information from schools. School Psychology Review, 31, 94–105.

Halle, J., Bambara, L. M., & Reichle, J. (2005). Teaching alternative skills. In L. M. Bambara & L. Kern (Eds.), Designing positive behavior supports for students (pp. 237–274). New York, NY: Guilford Press.

Hammen, C., Burge, D., & Stansbury, K. (1990). Relationship of mother and child variables to child outcomes in a high-risk sample: A causal modeling analysis. Developmental Psychology, 26, 24–30. doi:10.1037/0012-1649.26.1.24

Hancock, T. B., Kaiser, A. B., & Delaney, E. M. (2002). Teaching parents of preschoolers at high risk: Strategies to support language and positive behavior. Topics in Early Childhood Special Education, 22, 191–212. doi:10.1177/027112140202200402

Harry, B. (1992). Cultural diversity, families, and the special education system: Communication and empowerment. New York, NY: Teacher College Press.

Harry, B. (2002). Trends and issues in serving culturally diverse families of children with disabilities. Journal of Special Education. 36, 131–38, 47.

Hart, B., & Risley, R. T. (1995). Meaningful differences in the everyday experience of young American children. Baltimore, MD: Brookes.

Hartman, R. R., Stage, S. A., & Webster-Stratton, C. (2003). A growth curve analysis of parent training outcomes: Examining the influence of child risk factors (inattention, impulsivity, and hyperactivity problems), parental and family risk factors. Journal of Child Psychology and Psychiatry, and Allied Disciplines, 44, 388–398. doi:10.1111/1469-7610.00129

Hartsough, C. S., & Lambert, N. M. (1985). Medical factors in hyperactive and normal children: Prenatal, developmental, and health history findings. American Journal of Orthopsychiatry, 55, 190–201. doi:10.1111/j.1939-0025.1985.tb03433.x

Hawken, L. S., MacLeod, K. S., & Rawlings, L. (2007). Effects of the Behavior Education Program (BEP) on office discipline referrals of elementary school students. Journal of Positive Behavior Interventions, 9, 94–101. doi:10.1177/10983007070090020601

Hawkins, J. D., Catalano, R. F., & Miller, Y. (1992). Risk and protective factors for alcohol and other drug problems in adolescence and early adulthood: Implications for substance abuse prevention. Psychological Bulletin, 112, 64–105. doi:10.1037/0033-2909.112.1.64

Healey, D. M., Miller, C. J., Castelli, K. L., Marks, D. J., & Halperin, J. M. (2008). The impact of impairment criteria on rates of ADHD diagnoses in preschoolers. Journal of Abnormal Child Psychology, 36, 771–778. doi:10.1007/s10802-007-9209-1

Heffron, M. C., Grunstein, S., & Tilmon, S. (2007). Exploring diversity in supervision and practice. *Zero to Three, 28*(2), 34–38.

Hemeter, M. L., Corso, R., & Cheatham, R. (2006, February). *Issues in addressing challenging behavior in young children: A national survey of early childhood educators*. Presented at the Conference on Research Innovations in Early Intervention, San Diego, CA.

Hepburn, K. S. (2006). *Building culturally and linguistically competent services to support young children, their families, and school readiness*. Baltimore, MD: Annie E. Casey Foundation.

Herjanic, B., & Reich, W. (1982). Development of a structured psychiatric interview for children: Agreement between child and parent on individual symptoms. *Journal of Abnormal Child Psychology, 10*, 307–324.

Herring, S., Gray, K., Taffe, J., Tonge, B., Sweeney, D., & Einfeld, S. (2006). Behavior and emotional problems in toddlers with pervasive developmental disorders and developmental delay: Associations with parental mental health and family functioning. *Journal of Intellectual Disability Research, 50*, 874–882. doi:10.1111/j.1365-2788.2006.00904.x

Hinshaw, S. P., & Anderson, C. A. (1996). Conduct and oppositional defiant disorders. In R. A. Barkley & E. J. Mash (Eds.), *Child psychopathology* (pp. 113–149). New York, NY: Guilford Press.

Hoarea, P., & Beattie, T. (2003). Children with attention deficit hyperactivity disorder and attendance at hospital. *European Journal of Emergency Medicine, 10*, 98–100. doi:10.1097/00063110-200306000-00005

Hojnoski, R. L., Silberglitt, B., & Floyd, R. G. (2009). Sensitivity to growth over time of the Preschool Numeracy Indicators with a sample of preschoolers in Head Start. *School Psychology Review, 38*, 402–418.

Horner, R. H., Sugai, G., Todd, A. W., & Lewis-Palmer, T. (2006). Schoolwide positive behavior support. In L. M. Bambara & L. Kern (Eds.), *Individualized supports for students with problem behaviors* (pp. 359–390). New York, NY: Guilford Press.

Hoskyn, M. (2009). The prevention science perspective: Early intervention research on literacy, mathematics, and social competence. In S. Rosenfield & V. Berninger (Eds.), *Implementing evidence-based academic interventions in school settings* (pp. 165–212). New York, NY: Oxford University Press.

Hulme, C., Hatcher, P. J., Nation, K., Brown, A., Adams, J., & Stuart, G. (2002). Phoneme awareness is a better predictor of early reading skills than onset-rime awareness. *Journal of Experimental Child Psychology, 82*, 2–28.

Ingber, S., & Dromi, E. (2010). Actual versus desired family-centered practice in early intervention for children with hearing loss. *Journal of Deaf Studies and Deaf Education, 15*, 59–71. doi:10.1093/deafed/enp025

Invernizzi, M., Sullivan, A., Meier, J., & Swank, L. (2004). *PALS: Phonological Awareness Literacy Screening Pre-K technical reference*. Charlottesville: University of Virginia.

Isaksen, S. G., Treffinger, D. J., & Dorval, K. B. (2000). *Creative approaches to problem solving: A framework for change.* Dubuque, IA: Kendall-Hunt.

Iwata, B. A., Dorsey, M. F., Slifer, K. J., Bauman, K. E., & Richman, G. S. (1982). Toward a functional analysis of self-injury. *Analysis and Intervention in Developmental Disabilities, 2,* 3–20. doi:10.1016/0270-4684(82)90003-9

Jacobson, N. S., & Truax, P. (1991). Clinical significance: A statistical approach to defining meaningful change in psychotherapy research. *Journal of Consulting and Clinical Psychology, 59,* 12–19. doi:10.1037/0022-006X.59.1.12

Janney, R., & Snell, M. E. (2000). *Teacher's guide to inclusive practices: Behavioral support.* Baltimore, MD: Brookes.

Jensen, P. S. (2004). *Making the system work for your child with ADHD.* New York, NY: Guilford Press.

Jimerson, S. R., Burns, M. K., & VanDerHeyden, A. M. (Eds.). (2007). *Handbook of response to intervention: The science and practice of assessment and intervention.* New York, NY: Springer.

Joe, J. R., & Malach, R. S. (1998). Families with Native American roots. In E. W. Lynch & M. J. Hanson (Eds.), *Developing cross-cultural competence: A guide for working with children and their families* (2nd ed., pp. 127–164). Baltimore, MD: Brookes.

Johnston, C., & Mash, E. J. (2001). Families of children with attention-deficit/hyperactivity disorder: Review and recommendations for future research. *Clinical Child and Family Psychology Review, 4,* 183–207. doi:10.1023/A:1017592030434

Jokela, M., Power, C., & Kivimäki, M. (2009). Childhood problem behaviors and injury risk over the life course. *Journal of Child Psychology and Psychiatry, and Allied Disciplines, 50,* 1541–1549. doi:10.1111/j.1469-7610.2009.02122.x

Juel, C. (1988). Learning to read and write: A longitudinal study of 54 children from first through fourth grades. *Journal of Educational Psychology, 80,* 437–447. doi:10.1037/0022-0663.80.4.437

Justice, L. M., Chow, S. M., Capellini, C., Flanigan, K., & Colton, S. (2003). Emergent literacy intervention for vulnerable preschoolers: Relative effects of two approaches. *American Journal of Speech-Language Pathology, 12,* 320–332.

Justice, L. M., Kaderavek, J. N., Xitao, F., Sofka, A., & Hunt, A. (2009). Accelerating preschoolers' early literacy development through classroom-based teacher–child storybook reading and explicit print referencing. *Language, Speech, and Hearing Services in Schools, 40,* 67–85.

Kame'enui, E. J. (1993). Diverse learners and the tyranny of time: Don't fix blame, fix the leaky roof. *The Reading Teacher, 46,* 376–383.

Kaminski, R. A., & Good, R. H. (1996). Toward a technology for assessing basic early literacy skills. *School Psychology Review, 25,* 215–227.

Kazdin, A. E. (2001). *Behavior modification in applied settings* (6th ed.). Belmont, CA: Wadsworth/Thomson Learning.

Keenan, K., Shaw, D., Walsh, B., Deliquadri, E., & Giovanelli, J. (1997). *DSM–III–R* disorders in preschool children from low-income families. *Journal of the American Academy of Child and Adolescent Psychiatry, 36,* 620–627. doi:10.1097/00004583-199705000-00012

Kellam, S. G., & Rebok, G. W. (1992). Building developmental and etiological theory through epidemiologically based preventive intervention trials. In J. McCord & R. E. Tremblay (Eds.), *Preventing antisocial behavior: Interventions from birth through adolescence* (pp. 162–195). New York, NY: Guilford Press.

Kennedy, C. H., & Meyer, K. A. (1996). Sleep deprivation, allergy symptoms, and negatively reinforced problem behavior. *Journal of Applied Behavior Analysis, 29,* 133–135. doi:10.1901/jaba.1996.29-133

Keown, L. J., & Woodward, L. J. (2002). Early parent–child relations and family functioning of preschool boys with pervasive hyperactivity. *Journal of Abnormal Child Psychology, 30,* 541–553. doi:10.1023/A:1020803412247

Kern, L., DuPaul, G. J., Volpe, R. J., Sokol, N. G., Lutz, J. G., Arbolino, L. A. . . . VanBrakle, J. D. (2007). Multisetting assessment-based intervention for young children at risk for attention deficit hyperactivity disorder: Initial effects on academic and behavioral functioning. *School Psychology Review, 36,* 237–255.

Kern, L., Hilt-Panahon, A., & Sokol, N. (2009). Further examining the triangle tip: Improving support for students with emotional and behavioral needs. *Psychology in the Schools, 46,* 18–32. doi:10.1002/pits.20351

Kern, L., O'Neill, R. E., & Starosta, K. (2005). Gathering functional assessment information. In L. M. Bambara & L. Kern (Eds.), *Individualized supports for students with problem behavior* (pp. 129–164). New York, NY: Guilford Press.

Kersh, J., Hedvat, T. T., Hauser-Cram, P., & Warfield, M. E. (2006). The contribution of marital quality to the well-being of parents of children with developmental disabilities. *Journal of Intellectual Disability Research, 50,* 883–893. doi:10.1111/j.1365-2788.2006.00906.x

Knoster, T., & Kincaid, D. (2005). Long-term supports and ongoing evaluation. In L. M. Bambara & L. Kern (Eds.), *Designing positive behavior supports for students* (pp. 303–333). New York, NY: Guilford Press.

Koegel, L. K., Koegel, R. L., Boettcher, M., & Brookman-Frazee, L. (2005). Extending behavior support in home and community settings. In L. M. Bambara & L. Kern (Eds.), *Designing positive behavior supports for students* (pp. 334–358). New York, NY: Guilford Press.

Koegel, R. L., Koegel, L. K., & Schreibman, L. (1991). Assessing and training parents in teaching pivotal behaviors. *Advances in Behavioral Assessment of Children and Families, 5,* 65–82.

Kollins, S. H., & Greenhill, L. (2006). Evidence based for the use of stimulant medication in preschool children with ADHD. *Infants and Young Children, 19,* 132–141. doi:10.1097/00001163-200604000-00006

Kollins, S., Greenhill, L., Swanson, J., Wigal, S., Abikoff, H., McCracken, J., . . . & Bauzo, A. (2006). Rationale, design, and methods of the Preschool ADHD

Treatment Study (PATS). *Journal of the American Academy of Child and Adolescent Psychiatry, 45*, 1275–1283. doi:10.1097/01.chi.0000235074.86919.dc

Koutsoftas, A. D., Harmon, M. T., & Gray, S. (2009). The effect of Tier 2 intervention for phonemic awareness in a response-to-intervention model in low-income preschool classrooms. *Language, Speech, and Hearing Services in Schools, 40*, 116–130. doi:10.1044/0161-1461(2008/07-0101)

Kratochwill, T. R., & Bergan, J. R. (1990). *Behavioral consultation in applied settings.* New York, NY: Plenum Press.

LaFasto, F., & Larson, C. (2001). *When teams work best: 6000 team members and leaders tell what it takes to succeed.* Thousand Oaks, CA: Sage.

Lahey, B. B. (2000, October). *Assessment issues in doing research with preschoolers.* Paper presented at the annual convention of the American Academy of Child and Adolescent Psychiatry (Research Forum), New York, NY.

Lahey, B. B., Hartung, C. M., Loney, J., Pelham, W. E., Chronis, A. M., & Lee, S. S. (2007). Are there sex differences in the predictive validity of *DSM–IV* ADHD among younger children? *Journal of Clinical Child and Adolescent Psychology, 36*, 113–126. doi:10.1080/15374410701274066

Lahey, B. B., & Loeber, R. (1997). Attention-deficit/hyperactivity disorder, oppositional defiant disorder, conduct disorder, and adult antisocial behavior: A life span perspective. In D. M. Stoff, J. Breiling, & J. D. Maser (Eds.), *Handbook of antisocial behavior* (pp. 51–59). New York, NY: Wiley.

Lahey, B. B., Pelham, W. E., Loney, J., Kipp, H., Ehrhardt, A., Lee, S. S., . . . Massetti, G. (2004). Three-year predictive validity of *DSM–IV* attention deficit hyperactivity disorder in children diagnosed at 4–6 years of age. *The American Journal of Psychiatry, 161*, 2014–2020. doi:10.1176/appi.ajp.161.11.2014

Lahey, B. B., Pelham, W. E., Stein, M. A., Loney, J., Trapani, C., Nugent, K., . . . & Baumann, B. (1998). Validity of *DSM–IV* attention-deficit/hyperactivity disorder for younger children. *Journal of the American Academy of Child and Adolescent Psychiatry, 37*, 695–702. doi:10.1097/00004583-199807000-00008

Lahey, B. B., Piacentini, J. C., McBurnett, K., Stone, P., Hartdagen, S., & Hynd, G. (1988). Psychopathology in the parents of children with conduct disorder and hyperactivity. *Journal of the American Academy of Child and Adolescent Psychiatry, 27*, 163–170. doi:10.1097/00004583-198803000-00005

Lavigne, J. V., Gibbons, R. D., Christoffel, K. K., Arend, R., Rosenbaum, D., Binns, H., . . . & Isaacs, C. (1996). Prevalence rates and correlates of psychiatric disorders among preschool children. *Journal of the American Academy of Child and Adolescent Psychiatry, 35*, 204–214. doi:10.1097/00004583-199602000-00014

Lavigne, J. V., LeBailly, S. A., Hopkins, J., Gouze, K. R., & Binns, H. J. (2009). The prevalence of ADHD, ODD, depression, and anxiety in a community sample of 4-year-olds. *Journal of Clinical Child and Adolescent Psychology, 38*, 315–328. doi:10.1080/15374410902851382

Lee, S. S., Harrington, R. A., Chang, J. J., & Connors, S. L. (2008). Increased risk of injury in children with developmental disabilities. *Research in Developmental Disabilities, 29*, 247–255.

Lee, S. S., Lahey, B. B., Owens, E. B., & Hinshaw, S. P. (2008). Few preschool boys and girls with ADHD are well-adjusted during adolescence. *Journal of Abnormal Child Psychology, 36,* 373–383. doi:10.1007/s10802-007-9184-6

Levenstein, P. (1992). The mother–child home program: Research methodology and the real world. In J. McCord & R. E. Tremblay (Eds.), *Preventing antisocial behavior: Interventions from birth through adolescence* (pp. 43–66). New York, NY: Guilford Press.

Lewis, T. J., Sugai, G., & Colvin, G. (1998). Reducing problem behavior through a school-wide system of effective behavioral support: Investigation of a school-wide social skills training program and contextual interventions. *School Psychology Review, 27,* 446–459.

Loeber, R., Green, S. M., Keenan, K., & Lahey, B. B. (1995). Which boys will fare worse? Early predictors of the onset of conduct disorder in a six-year longitudinal study. *Journal of the American Academy of Child and Adolescent Psychiatry, 34,* 499–509. doi:10.1097/00004583-199504000-00017

Lonigan, C. J., Driscoll, K., Phillips, B. M., Cantor, B. G., Anthony, J. L., & Goldstein, H. (2003). A computer-assisted instruction phonological sensitivity program for preschool children at-risk for reading problems. *Journal of Early Intervention, 25,* 248–262.

Loughran, S. B. (2003). Agreement and stability of teacher rating scales for assessing ADHD in preschoolers. *Early Childhood Education Journal, 30,* 247–253.

Lucyshyn, J. M., & Albin, R. W. (1993). Comprehensive support to families of children with disabilities and problem behaviors: Keeping it "friendly." In G. H. S. Singer & L. E. Powers (Eds.), *Families, disability, and empowerment: Active coping skills and strategies for family interventions* (pp. 365–407). Baltimore, MD: Brookes.

Lucyshyn, J. M., Horner, R. H., Dunlap, G., Albin, R. W., & Ben, K. (2002). Positive behavior support with families. In J. M. Lucyshyn, G. Dunlap, & R. W. Albin (Eds.), *Families and positive behavior support* (pp. 3–43). Baltimore, MD: Brookes.

Lustig, D. C. (2002). Family coping in families with a child with a disability. *Education and Training in Mental Retardation and Developmental Disabilities, 37,* 14–22.

Luthar, S. S., & Zelazo, L. B. (2003). Research on resilience: An integrative review. In S. S. Luthar (Ed.), *Resilience and vulnerability: Adaptation in the context of childhood adversities* (pp. 510–550). New York, NY: Cambridge University Press. doi:10.1017/CBO9780511615788.023

Lynch, E. W., & Hanson, M. J. (2004). *Developing cross-cultural competence: A guide for working with children and their families* (3rd ed.). Baltimore, MD: Brookes.

Mahone, E. M., Pillion, J. P., & Hiemenz, J. R. (2001). Initial development of an auditory continuous performance test for preschoolers. *Journal of Attention Disorders, 5,* 93–106. doi:10.1177/108705470100500203

Mahone, E. M., Pillion, J. P., Hoffman, J., Hiemenz, J. R., & Denckla, M. B. (2005). Construct validity of the Auditory Continuous Performance Test for Preschoolers. *Developmental Neuropsychology, 27,* 11–33. doi:10.1207/s15326942dn2701_2

Mangus, R. S., Bergman, D., Zieger, M., & Coleman, J. J. (2004). Burn injuries in children with attention-deficit/hyperactivity disorder. *Burns, 30,* 148–150. doi: 10.1016/j.burns.2003.09.020

Maniadaki, K., Sonuga-Barke, E., Kakouros, E., & Karaba, R. (2007). Parental beliefs about the nature of ADHD behaviours and their relationship to referral intentions in preschool children. *Child: Care, Health and Development, 33,* 188–195.

Mariani, M., & Barkley, R. A. (1997). Neuropsychological and academic functioning in preschool children with attention deficit hyperactivity disorder. *Developmental Neuropsychology, 13,* 111–129. doi:10.1080/87565649709540671

Marks, D. J., Mlodnicka, A., Bernstein, M., Chacko, A., Rose, S., & Halperin, J. M. (2009). Profiles of service utilization and the resultant economic impact in preschoolers with attention deficit/hyperactivity disorder. *Journal of Pediatric Psychology, 34,* 681–689. doi:10.1093/jpepsy/jsn112

Mash, E. J., & Johnston, C. (1982). A comparison of the mother–child interactions of younger and older hyperactive and normal children. *Child Development, 53,* 1371–1381. doi:10.2307/1129028

Massetti, G. M., Lahey, B. B., Pelham, W. E., Loney, J., Ehrhardt, A., Lee, S. S., & Kip, H. (2008). Academic achievement over 8 years among children who met modified criteria for attention-deficit/hyperactivity disorder at 4–6 years of age. *Journal of Abnormal Child Psychology, 36,* 399–410. doi:10.1007/s10802-007-9186-4

Mayer, G. R., & Butterworth, T. W. (1979). A preventive approach to school violence and vandalism: An experimental study. *The Personnel and Guidance Journal, 57,* 436–441.

McGee, R., Partridge, F., Williams, S., & Silva, P. A. (1991). A twelve-year follow-up of preschool hyperactive children. *Journal of the American Academy of Child and Adolescent Psychiatry, 30,* 224–232. doi:10.1097/00004583-199103000-00010

McGill-Franzen, A. (1987). Failure to learn to read: Formulating a policy problem. *Reading Research Quarterly, 22,* 475–490. doi:10.2307/747703

McGoey, K. E., DuPaul, G. J., Eckert, T. L., Volpe, R. J., & Van Brakle, J. (2005). Outcomes of a multi-component intervention for preschool children at-risk for attention-deficit/hyperactivity disorder. *Child & Family Behavior Therapy, 27,* 33–56. doi:10.1300/J019v27n01_03

McGoey, K. E., DuPaul, G. J., Haley, E., & Shelton, T. L. (2007). Parent and teacher ratings of attention-deficit/hyperactivity disorder in preschool: The ADHD Rating Scale—IV Preschool Version. *Journal of Psychopathology and Behavioral Assessment, 29,* 269–276. doi:10.1007/s10862-007-9048-y

McGoey, K. E., Eckert, T. L., & DuPaul, G. J. (2002). Intervention for preschool-aged children with ADHD: A literature review. *Journal of Emotional and Behavioral Disorders, 10,* 14–28. doi:10.1177/106342660201000103

McNamara, K., Dennis, A. R., & Carte, T. A. (2008). It's the thought that counts: The mediating effects of information processing in virtual team decision making. *Information Systems Management, 25,* 20–32. doi:10.1080/10580530701777123

Michael, J. (1993). Establishing operations. *The Behavior Analyst, 16*, 191–206.

Milich, R., Landau, S., Kilby, G., & Whitten, P. (1982). Preschool peer perceptions of the behavior of hyperactive and aggressive children. *Journal of Abnormal Child Psychology, 10*, 497–510. doi:10.1007/BF00920750

Miltenberger, R. G. (2005). Strategies for measuring behavior change. In L. M. Bambara & L. Kern (Eds.), *Individualized supports for students with problem behavior* (pp. 107–128). New York, NY: Guilford Press.

Mitchell, E. A., Aman, M. G., Turbott, S. H., & Manku, M. (1987). Clinical characteristics and serum essential fatty acid levels in hyperactive children. *Clinical Pediatrics, 26*, 406–411.

Molina, B. S. G., Hinshaw, S. P., Swanson, J. M., Arnold, L. E., Vitiello, B., Jensen, P. S., . . . & the MTA Cooperative Group. (2009). MTA at 8 years: Prospective follow-up of children treated for combined-type ADHD in a multisite study. *Journal of the American Academy of Child and Adolescent Psychiatry, 48*, 484–500. doi:10.1097/CHI.0b013e31819c23d0

Mortenson, B. P., & Witt, J. C. (1998). The use of weekly performance feedback to increase teacher implementation of a prereferral academic intervention. *School Psychology Review, 27*, 613–627.

MTA Cooperative Group. (1999). A 14-month randomized clinical trial of treatment strategies for attention-deficit/hyperactivity disorder. *Archives of General Psychiatry, 56*, 1073–1086. doi:10.1001/archpsyc.56.12.1073

MTA Cooperative Group. (2004). The NIMH MTA follow-up: 24-month outcomes of treatment strategies for attention-deficit/hyperactivity disorder (ADHD). *Pediatrics, 113*, 754–761. doi:10.1542/peds.113.4.754

Müller, E. (February, 2007). *Statewide behavior initiatives*. Alexandria, VA: Forum Project, National Association of State Directors of Special Education.

Murray, D. W., Kollins, S. H., Hardy, K. K., Abikoff, H. B., Swanson, J. M., Cunningham, C., . . . & Chuang, S. Z. (2007). Parent versus teacher ratings of attention-deficit/hyperactivity disorder in the Preschoolers with Attention-Deficit/Hyperactivity Disorder Treatment Study (PATS). *Journal of Child and Adolescent Psychopharmacology, 17*, 605–619. doi:10.1089/cap.2007.0060

National Reading Panel. (2000). *Teaching children to read: An evidence-based assessment of the scientific research literature on reading and its implications for reading instruction: Reports of the subgroups*. Bethesda, MD: National Institute of Child Health and Human Development.

Neely-Barnes, S., & Dia, D. A. (2008). Families of children with disabilities: A review of the literature and recommendations for interventions. *Journal of Early and Intensive Behavior Intervention, 5*, 93–107.

Newborg, J., Stock, J. R., & Wnek, L. (1988). *Manual for the Battelle Developmental Inventory*. Boston, MA: Houghton Mifflin.

Nigg, J. T. (2006). *What causes ADHD?* New York, NY: Guilford Press.

Nigg, J. T., & Hinshaw, S. P. (1998). Parent personality traits and psychopathology associated with antisocial behaviors in childhood attention-deficit hyperactivity disorder. *Journal of Child Psychology and Psychiatry, and Allied Disciplines, 39*, 145–159. doi:10.1017/S0021963097001984

Noell, G. H., Witt, J. C., Gilbertson, D. N., Ranier, D. D., & Freeland, J. T. (1997). Increasing teacher intervention implementation in general education settings through consultation and performance feedback. *School Psychology Quarterly, 12*, 77–88. doi:10.1037/h0088949

Northup, J., Fusilier, I., Swanson, V., Huete, J., Bruce, T., Freeland, J., . . . & Edwards, S. (1999). Further analysis of the separate and interactive effects of methylphenidate and common classroom contingencies. *Journal of Applied Behavior Analysis, 32*, 35–50. doi:10.1901/jaba.1999.32-35

Northup, J., Jones, K., Broussard, C., DiGiovanni, G., Herring, M., Fusilier, I., & Hanchey, A. (1997). A preliminary analysis of interactive effects between common classroom contingencies and methylphenidate. *Journal of Applied Behavior Analysis, 30*, 121–125. doi:10.1901/jaba.1997.30-121

Northup, J., Wacker, D., Sasso, G., Steege, M., Cigrand, K., Cook, J., & DeRaad, A. (1991). A brief functional analysis of aggressive and alternative behavior in an outclinic setting. *Journal of Applied Behavior Analysis, 24*, 509–522. doi:10.1901/jaba.1991.24-509

Notari-Syverson, A., O'Connor, R. E., & Vadasy, P. F. (1998). *Ladders to Literacy: A preschool activity book*. Baltimore, MD: Brookes.

Offord, D. R., Boyle, M. H., & Racine, Y. A. (1991). The epidemiology of antisocial behavior in childhood and adolescence. In D. J. Pepler & K. H. Rubin (Eds.), *The development and treatment of childhood aggression* (pp. 31–54). Hillsdale, NJ: Erlbaum.

O'Neill, R. E., Horner, R. H., Albin, R. W., Sprague, J. R., Storey, K., & Newton, J. (1997). *Functional assessment and program development for problem behavior: A practical handbook* (2nd ed.). Pacific Grove, CA: Sopris West.

O'Reilly, M. (2002). *Early literacy skill development of kindergartners and first-graders at-risk for externalizing behavior disorders*. Unpublished manuscript, University of Massachusetts Amherst.

Orvaschel, H., & Puig-Antich, J. (1994). *The Kiddie—SADS—E* (5th revision). Ft. Lauderdale, FL: Center for Psychological Studies, Nova Southeastern University.

Patterson, G. R. (1982). *Coercive family process*. Eugene, OR: Castalia.

Patterson, G. (1995). Coercion as a basis for early age of onset for arrest. In J. McCord (Ed.), *Coercion and punishment in long-term perspectives* (pp. 81–105). New York, NY: Cambridge University Press.

Patterson, G. R., Reid, J. B., & Dishion, T. J. (1992). *Antisocial boys*. Eugene, OR: Castalia.

Pelham, W. E., Jr., & Fabiano, G. A. (2008). Evidence-based psychosocial treatments for attention-deficit/hyperactivity disorder. *Journal of Clinical Child and Adolescent Psychology, 37,* 184–214. doi:10.1080/15374410701818681

Pelham, W. E., Jr., Fabiano, G. A., & Massetti, G. M. (2005). Evidence-based assessment of attention deficit hyperactivity disorder in children and adolescents. *Journal of Clinical Child and Adolescent Psychology, 34,* 449–476. doi:10.1207/s15374424jccp3403_5

Pelham, W. E., Foster, E. M., & Robb, J. A. (2007). Economic impact of attention-deficit/hyperactivity disorder in children and adolescents. *Journal of Pediatric Psychology, 32,* 711–727. doi:10.1093/jpepsy/jsm022

Pelham, W. E., Gnagy, E. M., Greenslade, K. E., & Milich, R. (1992). Teacher ratings of *DSM–III–R* symptoms for the disruptive behavior disorders. *Journal of the American Academy of Child and Adolescent Psychiatry, 31,* 210–218. doi:10.1097/00004583-199203000-00005

Peterson, C., Jesso, B., & McCabe, A. (1999). Encouraging narratives in preschoolers: An intervention study. *Journal of Child Language, 26,* 49–67. doi:10.1017/S0305000998003651

Phaneuf, R. L., & Silberglitt, B. (2003). Tracking preschoolers' language and preliteracy development using a general outcome measurement system: One education district's experience. *Topics in Early Childhood Special Education, 23,* 114–123.

Phillips, P. L., Greenson, J. N., Collett, B. R., & Gimpel, G. A. (2002). Assessing ADHD symptoms in preschool children: Use of the ADHD symptoms rating scale. *Early Education and Development, 13,* 283–300. doi:10.1207/s15566935eed1303_3

Pierce, E. W., Ewing, L. J., & Campbell, S. B. (1999). Diagnostic status and symptomatic behavior of hard-to-manage preschool children in middle childhood and early adolescence. *Journal of Clinical Child Psychology, 28,* 44–57. doi:10.1207/s15374424jccp2801_4

Power, T. J., DuPaul, G. J., Shapiro, E. S., & Kazak, A. E. (2003). *Promoting children's health: Integrating school, family, and community.* New York, NY: Guilford Press.

Premack, D. (1959). Toward empirical behavioral laws: I. Positive reinforcement. *Psychological Review, 66,* 219–233. doi:10.1037/h0040891

Primavera, J. (2000). Enhancing family competence through literacy activities. *Journal of Prevention & Intervention in the Community, 20,* 85–101.

Purpura, D. J., & Lonigan, C. J. (2009). Conners' Teacher Rating Scale for preschool children: A revised, brief, age-specific measure. *Journal of Clinical Child and Adolescent Psychology, 38,* 263–272. doi:10.1080/15374410802698446

Rappley, M. D. (2006). Actual psychotropic medication use in preschool children. *Infants and Young Children, 19,* 154–163. doi:10.1097/00001163-200604000-00008

Rappley, M. D., Eneli, I. U., Mullan, P. B., Alvarez, F. J., Wang, J., Luo, Z., & Gardiner, J. C. (2002). Patterns of psychotropic medication use in very young children with attention-deficit hyperactivity disorder. *Developmental and Behavioral Pediatrics, 23,* 23–30.

Rapport, M. D., Alderson, R. M., Kofler, M. J., Sarver, D. E., Bolden, J., & Sims, V. (2008). Working memory deficits in boys with attention-deficit/hyperactivity disorder (ADHD): The contribution of central executive and subsystem processes. *Journal of Abnormal Child Psychology, 36*, 825–837. doi:10.1007/s10802-008-9215-y

Rapport, M. D., Denney, C. B., DuPaul, G. J., & Gardner, M. J. (1994). Attention deficit disorder and methylphenidate: Normalization rates, clinical effectiveness, and response prediction in 76 children. *Journal of the American Academy of Child and Adolescent Psychiatry, 33*, 882–893. doi:10.1097/00004583-199407000-00015

Reid, J. B., & Eddy, J. M. (1997). The prevention of antisocial behavior: Some considerations in the search for effective interventions. In D. M. Stoff, J. Breiling, & J. D. Maser (Eds.), *Handbook of antisocial behavior* (pp. 343–356). New York, NY: Wiley.

Reid, R., Trout, A. L., & Schartz, M. (2005). Self-regulation interventions for children with attention deficit/hyperactivity disorder. *Exceptional Children, 71*, 361–377.

Reynolds, C. R., & Kamphaus, R. W. (2002). *BASC–2: Behavioral Assessment System for Children* (2nd ed.). Upper Saddle River, NJ: Pearson.

Robins, D. L., Fein, D., Barton, M. L., & Green, J. A. (2001). The Modified Checklist for Autism in Toddlers: An initial study investigating the early detection of autism and pervasive developmental disorders. *Journal of Autism and Developmental Disorders, 31*, 131–144.

Robinson, K. A., Dennison, C. R., Wayman, D. M., Pronovost, P. J., & Needham, D. M. (2007). Systematic review identifies number of strategies important for retaining study participants. *Journal of Clinical Epidemiology, 60*, 757–765. doi:10.1016/j.jclinepi.2006.11.023

Rock, M. L., & Thead, B. K. (2007). The effects of fading a strategic self-monitoring intervention on students' academic engagement, accuracy, and productivity. *Journal of Behavioral Education, 16*, 389–412. doi:10.1007/s10864-007-9049-7

Rowe, R., Maughan, B., & Goodman, R. (2004). Childhood psychiatric disorder and unintentional injury: Findings from a national cohort study. *Journal of Pediatric Psychology, 29*, 119–130. doi:10.1093/jpepsy/jsh015

Rushton, J. L., & Whitmire, J. T. (2001). Pediatric stimulant and selective serotonin reuptake inhibitor prescription trends: 1992 to 1998. *Archives of Pediatrics & Adolescent Medicine, 155*, 560–565.

Rutter, M. (1997). Antisocial behavior: Developmental psychopathology perspectives. In D. M. Stoff, J. Breiling, & J. D. Maser (Eds.), *Handbook of antisocial behavior* (pp. 115–124). New York, NY: Wiley.

Sasso, G. M., Conroy, M. A., Stichter, J. P., & Fox, J. P. (2001). Slowing down the bandwagon: The misapplication of functional assessment for students with emotional or behavioral disorders. *Behavioral Disorders, 26*, 282–296.

Schippers, A., & van Boheemen, M. (2009). Family quality of life empowered by family-oriented support. *Journal of Policy and Practice in Intellectual Disabilities, 6,* 19–24. doi:10.1111/j.1741-1130.2008.00195.x

Schwebel, D. C., Brezausek, C. M., Ramey, S. L., & Ramey, C. T. (2004). Interactions between child behavior patterns and parenting: Implications for children's unintentional injury risk. *Journal of Pediatric Psychology, 29,* 93–104. doi:10.1093/jpepsy/jsh013

Schwebel, D. C., Speltz, M. L., Jones, K., & Bardina, P. (2002). Unintentional injury in preschool boys with and without early onset of disruptive behavior. *Journal of Pediatric Psychology, 27,* 727–737. doi:10.1093/jpepsy/27.8.727

Shaffer, D., Fisher, P., Lucas, C., Dulcan, M., & Schwab-Stone, M. (2000). NIMH Diagnostic Interview Schedule for Children Version IV (NIMH DISC–IV): Description, differences from previous versions, and reliability of some common diagnoses. *Journal of the American Academy of Child and Adolescent Psychiatry, 39,* 28–38. doi:10.1097/00004583-200001000-00014

Shapiro, E. S. (2004). *Academic skills problems: Direct assessment and intervention* (3rd ed.). New York, NY: Guilford Press.

Shelton, T. L., Barkley, R. A., Crosswait, C., Moorehouse, M., Fletcher, K., Barret, S., . . . & Metevia, L. (1998). Psychiatric and psychological morbidity as a function of adaptive disability in preschool children with aggressive and hyperactive-impulsive-inattentive behavior. *Journal of Abnormal Child Psychology, 26,* 475–494. doi:10.1023/A:1022603902905

Shinn, M. R. (Ed.). (1998). *Advanced applications of curriculum-based measurement.* New York, NY: Guilford Press.

Simmerman, S., Blacher, J., & Baker, B. L. (2001) Fathers' and mothers' perceptions of father involvement in families with young children with a disability. *Journal of Intellectual and Developmental Disability, 26, 4,* 325–338.

Singer, G. H. S., & Irvin, L. K. (1991). Supporting families of persons with severe disabilities: Emerging findings, practices, and questions. In H. H. Meyer, C. A. Peck, & L. Brown (Eds.), *Critical issues in the lives of people with severe disabilities* (pp. 271–312). Baltimore, MD: Brookes.

Singh, I. (2003). Boys will be boys: Father's perspectives on ADHD symptoms, diagnosis, and drug treatment. *Harvard Review of Psychiatry, 11,* 308–316.

Sinkovits, H. S., Kelly, M., & Ernst, M. (2003). Medication administration in day care centers for children. *Journal of the American Pharmacists Association, 43,* 379–382. doi:10.1331/154434503321831094

Skinner, B. F. (1953). *Science and human behavior.* New York, NY: Macmillan.

Smith, K. G., & Corkum, P. (2007). Systematic review of measurers used to diagnose attention-deficit/hyperactivity disorder in research on preschool children. *Topics in Early Childhood Special Education, 27,* 164–173.

Snell, M. E., & Janney, R. E. (2000). Teachers' problem-solving about children with moderate and severe disabilities in elementary classrooms. *Exceptional Children, 66,* 472–490.

Snow, C. E., Burns, S., & Griffin, P. (Eds.). (1998). *Preventing reading difficulties in young children*. Washington, DC: National Academies Press.

Sobol, M. P., Ashbourne, D. T., Earn, B. M., & Cunningham, C. E. (1989). Parents' attributions for achieving compliance from attention-deficit disordered children. *Journal of Abnormal Child Psychology, 17*, 359–369. doi:10.1007/BF00917405

Sokol, N. G. (2002). *Early numeracy skills assessment*. Unpublished manuscript, Lehigh University, Bethlehem, PA.

Sokol, N. G., Kern, L., Arbolino, L. A., Thomas, L. B., & DuPaul, G. J. (2009). A summary of home-based functional analysis data for young children with or at risk for attention-deficit/hyperactivity disorder. *Early Childhood Services: An Interdisciplinary Journal of Effectiveness, 3*, 127–142.

Sonuga-Barke, J. S., Auerbach, J., Campbell, S. B., Daley, D., & Thompson, M. (2005). Varieties of preschool hyperactivity: Multiple pathways from risk to disorder. *Developmental Science, 8*, 141–150.

Sonuga-Barke, E. J., Daley, D., Thompson, M., Laver-Bradbury, C., & Weeks, A. (2001). Parent-based therapies for preschool attention-deficit/hyperactivity disorder: A randomized, controlled trial with a community sample. *Journal of the American Academy of Child and Adolescent Psychiatry, 40*, 402–408. doi:10.1097/00004583-200104000-00008

Sonuga-Barke, E. J., & Halperin, J. M. (2010). Developmental phenotypes and causal pathways in attention deficit/hyperactivity disorder: Potential targets for early intervention? *Journal of Child Psychology and Psychiatry, and Allied Disciplines, 51*, 368–389. doi:10.1111/j.1469-7610.2009.02195.x

Spencer, T. J. (2006). Antidepressants and specific norepinephrine reuptake inhibitor treatments. In R. A. Barkley (Ed.), *Attention-deficit/hyperactivity disorder: A handbook for diagnosis and treatment* (3rd ed., pp. 648–657). New York, NY: Guilford Press.

Spira, E. G., & Fischel, J. E. (2005). The impact of preschool inattention, hyperactivity, and impulsivity on social and academic development: A review. *Journal of Child Psychology and Psychiatry, and Allied Disciplines, 46*, 755–773. doi:10.1111/j.1469-7610.2005.01466.x

Sterba, S., Egger, H. L., & Angold, A. (2007). Diagnostic specificity and nonspecificity in the dimensions of preschool psychopathology. *Journal of Child Psychology and Psychiatry, and Allied Disciplines, 48*, 1005–1013. doi:10.1111/j.1469-7610.2007.01770.x

Stiebel, D. (1999). Promoting augmentative communication during daily routines: A parent problem-solving intervention. *Journal of Positive Behavior Interventions, 1*, 159–169.

Stokes, T. (1992). Discrimination and generalization. *Journal of Applied Behavior Analysis, 25*, 429–432. doi:10.1901/jaba.1992.25-429

Storch, S. A., & Whitehurst, G. J. (2002). Oral language and code-related precursors to reading: Evidence from a longitudinal structural model. *Developmental Psychology, 38*, 934–947. doi:10.1037/0012-1649.38.6.934

Strain, P. S., Steele, P., Ellis, T., & Timm, M. A. (1982). Long-term effects of oppositional child treatment with mothers as therapists and therapist trainers. *Journal of Applied Behavior Analysis, 15*, 163–169.

Straka, E., & Bricker, D. (1996). Building a collaborative team. In D. Bricker & A. Wonderstrom (Eds.), *Preparing personnel to work with infants and young children and their families: A team approach* (pp. 321–345). Baltimore, MD: Brookes.

Sugai, G., & Horner, R. H. (2002). The evolution of discipline practices: School-wide positive behavior supports. *Child & Family Behavior Therapy, 24*, 23–50. doi:10.1300/J019v24n01_03

Sulzer-Azeroff, B., & Mayer, G. R. (1986). *Achieving educational excellence: Using behavioral strategies.* San Marcos, CA: Western Image.

Swanson, J., Greenhill, L., Wigal, T., Kollins, S., Stehli, A., Davies, M., . . . & Wigal, S. (2006). Stimulant-related reductions of growth rates in the PATS. *Journal of the American Academy of Child and Adolescent Psychiatry, 45*, 1304–1313. doi:10.1097/01.chi.0000235075.25038.5a

Sylva, J. A. (2005). Issues in early intervention: The impact of cultural diversity on service delivery in natural environments. *Multicultural Education, 13*(2), 26–29.

Szatmari, P., Offord, D. R., & Boyle, M. H. (1989). Correlates, associated impairments, and patterns of service utilization of children with attention deficit disorders: Findings from the Ontario Child Health Study. *Journal of Child Psychology and Psychiatry, and Allied Disciplines, 30*, 205–217. doi:10.1111/j.1469-7610.1989.tb00235.x

Tandon, M., Si, X., Beiden, A., & Luby, J. (2009). Attention-deficit/hyperactivity disorder in preschool children: An investigation of validate based on visual attention performance. *Journal of Child and Adolescent Psychopharmacology, 19*, 137–146. doi:10.1089/cap.2008.048

Taylor, E. A., Sandberg, S., Thorley, F., & Giles, S. (1991). *The epidemiology of childhood hyperactivity.* London, England: Oxford University Press.

Thomas, C. R., Ayoub, M., Rosenberg, L., Robert, R. S., & Meyer, W. J. (2004). Attention deficit hyperactivity disorder & pediatric burn injury: A preliminary retrospective study. *Burns, 30*, 221–223. doi:10.1016/j.burns.2003.10.013

Torgesen, J. K. (2000). Individual differences in response to early interventions in reading: The lingering problem of treatment resisters. *Learning Disabilities Research & Practice, 15*, 55–64.

Torgesen, J. K., Alexander, A. W., Wagner, R. K., Rashotte, C. A., Voeller, K. K. S., & Conway, T. (2001). Intensive remedial instruction for children with severe reading disabilities: Immediate and long-term outcomes from two instructional approaches. *Journal of Learning Disabilities, 34*, 33–58.

Torgesen, J. K., Wagner, R. K., Rashotte, C. A., Rose, E., Lindamood, P., Conway, T., & Garvan, C. (1999). Preventing reading failure in young children with phonological processing disabilities: Group and individual responses to instruction. *Journal of Educational Psychology, 91*, 1–15.

Tremblay, R. E., Vitaro, F., Bertrand, L., LeBlanc, M., Beauchesne, H., Boileau, H., & David, L. (1992). Parent and child training to prevent early onset of delinquency: The Montreal Longitudinal-Experimental Study. In J. McCord & R. E. Tremblay (Eds.), *Preventing antisocial behavior: Interventions from birth through adolescence* (pp. 117–138). New York, NY: Guilford Press.

Turnbull, A. P., & Turnbull, H. R. (2000). *Families, professional, and exceptionality: Collaborating for empowerment.* Upper Saddle River, NJ: Prentice Hall.

van Kleeck, A. (2008). Providing preschool foundations for later reading comprehension: The importance of and ideas for targeting inferencing in storybook-sharing interventions. *Psychology in the Schools, 45,* 627–643.

van Kleeck, A., Vander Woude, J., & Hammett, L. (2006). Fostering literal and inferential language skills in Head Start preschoolers with language impairment using scripted book-sharing discussions. *American Journal of Speech-Language Pathology, 15,* 85–95.

van Lier, P. A. C., van der Ende, J., Koot, H. M., & Verhulst, F. C. (2007). Which better predicts conduct problems? The relationship of trajectories of conduct problems with ODD and ADHD symptoms from childhood into adolescence. *Journal of Child Psychology and Psychiatry, and Allied Disciplines, 48,* 601–608. doi:10.1111/j.1469-7610.2006.01724.x

Vitiello, B., Abikoff, H. B., Chuang, S. Z., Kollins, S. H., McCracken, J. T., Riddle, M. A., . . . & Greenhill, L. L. (2007). Effectiveness of methylphenidate in the 10-month continuation phase of the Preschoolers with ADHD Treatment Study (PATS). *Journal of Child and Adolescent Psychopharmacology, 17,* 593–603. doi:10.1089/cap.2007.0058

Wagner, R. K., & Torgesen, J. K. (1987). The nature of phonological processing and its causal role in the acquisition of reading skills. *Psychological Bulletin, 101,* 192–212.

Weinger, S. (1999). Views of the child with retardation: Relationship to family functioning. *Family Therapy, 26,* 63–79.

Walker, H. M., Horner, R. H., Sugai, G., Bullis, M., Sprague, J. R., Bricker, D., . . . Kaufman, M. J. (1996). Integrated approaches to preventing patterns among school-age children and youth. *Journal of Emotional and Behavioral Disorders, 4,* 194–209. doi:10.1177/106342669600400401

Walker, H. M., Severson, H.H., & Feil, E.G. (1995). *Early Screening Project (ESP): A proven child-find success.* Longmont, CO: Sopris West.

Walter, H. J., Gouze, K., & Lim, K. G. (2006). Teachers' beliefs about mental health needs in inner city elementary schools. *Journal of the American Academy for Child and Adolescent Psychiatry, 45,* 61–68.

Watson, S. M. R., & Keith, K. D. (2002). Comparing the quality of life of school-age children with and without disabilities. *Mental Retardation, 40,* 304–312.

Watson, T. S., & Steege, M. W. (2003). *Conducting school-based functional behavioral assessment: A practitioner's guide.* New York, NY: Guilford Press.

Wehmeyer, M. L., & Schalock, R. L. (2001). Self-determination and quality of life: Implications for special education services and supports. *Focus on Exceptional Children, 33,* 1–16.

Weinger, S. (1999). Views of the child with retardation: Relationship to family functioning. *Family Therapy, 26,* 63–79.

West, J., Denton, K., & Germino-Hausken, E. (2000). *America's kindergarteners: Findings from the Early Childhood Longitudinal Study, Kindergarten Class of 1998–99, Fall, 1998* (NCES 2000-070). Washington, DC: US Department of Education, National Center for Educational Statistics.

Wigal, T., Greenhill, L., Chuang, S., McGough, J., Vitiello, B., Skrobala, A., . . . & Stehli, A. (2006). Safety and tolerability of methylphenidate in preschool children with ADHD. *Journal of the American Academy of Child and Adolescent Psychiatry, 45,* 1294-1303.

Williford, A. P., & Shelton, T. L. (2008). Using mental health consultation to decrease disruptive behaviors in preschoolers: Adapting an empirically-supported intervention. *Journal of Child Psychology and Psychiatry, 49,* 191–200.

Wolraich, M. L. (2006). Attention-deficit/hyperactivity disorder: Can it be recognized and treated in children younger than 5 years? *Infants & Young Children, 19,* 86–93.

Woodcock, R. W., McGrew, K. S., & Mather, N. (2001). *Woodcock–Johnson III Tests of Achievement.* Itasca, IL: Riverside.

Zevenbergen, A., & Whitehurst, G. (2003). Dialogic reading: A shared picture book reading intervention for preschoolers. In A. van Kleeck, S. A. Stahl, & E. Bauer (Eds.), *On reading to children: Parents and teachers* (pp. 177–200). Mahwah, NJ: Erlbaum.

Zito, J. M., Safer, D. J., DosReis, S., Gardner, J. F., Boles, M., & Lynch, F. (2000). Trends in the prescribing of psychotropic medications to preschoolers. *JAMA, 283,* 1025–1030.

Zito, J. M., Safer, D. J., Valluri, S., Gardner, J. F., Korelitz, J. J., & Mattison, R. E. (2007). Psychotherapeutic medication prevalence in Medicaid-insured preschoolers. *Journal of Child and Adolescent Psychopharmacology, 17,* 195–203.

# INDEX

229

Diagnosis, *continued*
    challenges with, 38–40
    difficulties with, 5
    *DSM* criteria for, 53
    and early symptoms, 193
    need for early, 4
*Diagnostic and Statistical Manual of*
    *Mental Disorders* (4th ed., text
    revision; *DSM–IV–TR*)
    ADHD diagnosis, 53
    ADHD symptoms, 4–5, 7, 151, 187,
    192, 195
    and assessment, 23, 25, 26, 29, 34–36,
    46
    oppositional defiant disorder criteria,
    189
Diagnostic Interview for Children
    Version IV (DISC–IV), 27, 28
Diagnostic interviews
    for early intervention, 193
    for identifying alternative/comorbid
    disorders, 33, 36–37
    with parents, 27–28, 33
Dialogic reading. *See* Shared book reading
Direct observation. *See* Observation
DISC–IV (Diagnostic Interview for
    Children Version IV), 27, 28
Disruptive behavior(s)
    of adolescents, 13
    and assessment, 27–28
    in child-care settings, 11
    classifying behaviors as, 59
    and home-based intervention, 73
    observation of, 159
    and preschool-based intervention, 95
Disruptive behavior disorders, 129, 130
Distal events, 76, 98
Distracting behaviors
    classifying behaviors as, 59
    and home-based intervention, 73
    and preschool-based intervention, 95
Dopamine, 16
Dosage, of psychotropic medication,
    160, 161
*DSM–IV–TR. See Diagnostic and Statisti-*
    *cal Manual of Mental Disorders*
Dunlap, G., 169
DuPaul, G. J., 12, 103, 172
Dynamic Indicators of Basic Early Liter-
    acy Skills, 34

Early Childhood Home Observation for
    Measurement of the Environment
    (EC-HOME), 139
Early Childhood Inventory—4, 29
Early Intervention for ADHD (EIA)
    project, 186
Early intervention model, 185–201. *See*
    *also* Intervention
    areas of focus in, 194–195
    for cross-setting interventions,
    195–196
    early assessment and identification
    in, 192–193
    future directions for research,
    197–200
    and medication use, 185–187, 189,
    196–198
    outcome studies on, 185–192
    overview, 48–49
    potential outcomes with, 193–194
Early language skills, 109–112
Early mathematics skills, 46, 70,
    117–120
Early Numeracy Skills Assessment, 34
Early reading skills, 46, 113–117
Early Screening Project (ESP), 30, 31
EC-HOME (Early Childhood Home
    Observation for Measurement of
    the Environment), 139
Eckert, T. L., 103
Education, parent. *See* Parent education
Educational interventions, 43. *See also*
    Parent education
Educational services, 180
Egger, H. L., 5, 191
EIA (Early Intervention for ADHD)
    project, 186
Elementary school children, 13, 14, 23,
    198
Elliott, J., 122
Emotional problems, 88
Environmental factors, 15, 16, 23,
    37–38, 194. *See also* Home
    environment
ESP (Early Screening Project), 30, 31
Establishing operations. *See* Setting
    events
Executive functions, 16
Externalizing behavior problems, 18
Externalizing disorders, 29, 33

Parent–child interactions, *continued*
  patterns of, 55
  and psychiatric disorders, 174
Parent education
  for advocating for child services, 180
  group-based, 55, 64–71
  in home-based tiered model, 53–56
  for injury prevention, 131–137
  outcomes of treatment using,
    187–191
  for promoting child's language skills,
    110, 112
  for promoting child's mathematics
    skills, 118–119
Parent empowerment, 177–178
Parent-implemented intervention, 167.
    *See also* Home-based intervention
Parenting, cultural approaches to, 176,
  179
Parent ratings
  correlation between teacher ratings
    and, 37, 39
  of functional impairment, 33
  precedence of teacher ratings over,
    35, 36
  and symptom severity, 155
  tallying symptom counts from, 34
Partnerships, 58, 168–171
PATS. *See* Preschool ADHD Treatment
  Study
Patterson, G. R., 10, 63
Pedestrian accidents, 133, 136
Pediatricians, 158, 180
Peer relations. *See also* Social functioning
  of adolescents, 13
  assessment of, 34
  and disruptive behaviors, 11
  and intervention, 52
  and problem behavior, 97
Pelham, W. E., 15
Peterson, C., 112
Pharmacotherapy, 149, 198. *See also*
  Psychotropic medication
Phonemic awareness, 11, 116, 121, 122
Phonological awareness, 115–117
Phonological Awareness Literacy
  Screening, 34
Physical injuries. *See* Injuries
Physicians, 158
Play, 121

Poisonings, accidental, 12, 128–129,
    133, 134, 142–146, 195
Positive reinforcement, 75
Praise, 67
Preacademic skills, 10, 36, 50, 52, 189,
    194–195. *See also* Academic func-
    tioning
Premack principle, 68
Prereading skills, 13, 70, 108. *See also*
    Reading skills
Preschool ADHD Treatment Study
    (PATS), 6, 18, 151–153,
    186–187, 196
Preschool-age children
  ADHD symptoms in, 13, 14
  prevalence of ADHD in, 5, 6
  school services for, 15
Preschool-based intervention, 87–106
  assessment in, 90, 95–102
  case example, 103–105
  challenges with, 106
  and collaboration, 58
  evaluating progress in, 102–103
  obtaining buy-in in, 90–91
  overview, 56–58
  for preventing injuries, 131
  small-group skills instruction in, 89,
    90, 93–95
  tiered model of, 56–58, 88–101
  universal intervention in, 89–93
Preschool Numeracy Indicators, 34
Preschool settings
  and assessment, 28, 30, 31, 35
  delayed infrequent reinforcement in,
    17
  disruptive behavior in, 11
  and early intervention, 195
  injury prevention in, 137–138
  intervention in. *See* Preschool-based
    intervention
  and language skills, 110
  literacy environments in, 115, 116
  structured experiences in, 18
Prevention
  injury. *See* Injury prevention
  levels of, in tiered model, 19–20
Primary prevention, 19
Primavera, J., 114
Prior, M., 122
Problem behavior. *See* Behavior problems

# ABOUT THE AUTHORS

**George J. DuPaul, PhD,** is a professor of school psychology and chairperson of education and human services at Lehigh University, Bethlehem, Pennsylvania. He received his PhD in school psychology from the University of Rhode Island in 1985. He has extensive experience providing clinical services to children with attention-deficit/hyperactivity disorder (ADHD) and their families as well as consulting with a variety of school districts regarding the management of students with ADHD. He has been an author or coauthor on more than 160 journal articles and book chapters related to ADHD and childhood behavior disorders. He has published three books and produced two videos on the assessment and treatment of ADHD as well as two books related to children's health care. Dr. DuPaul was named to the Children and Adults with ADHD Hall of Fame in 2008 and also received the American Psychological Association Division 16 (School Psychology) Senior Scientist Award in 2008. Currently, he is investigating the effects of early intervention and school-based interventions for students with ADHD as well as assessment and treatment of ADHD in college students.

**Lee Kern, PhD,** is Iacocca Professor of Special Education at Lehigh University, Bethlehem, Pennsylvania. She received her PhD in special education from the University of South Florida. Prior to receiving her doctorate, Dr. Kern worked in the field of special education as a classroom teacher, behavior specialist, and consultant. She has worked extensively with children and adolescents with social, emotional, and behavioral problems. Her research interests include challenging behavior, functional assessment, and curricular interventions. She has published numerous articles and book chapters, and she recently published the book *Individualized Supports for Students With Problem Behaviors*. Dr. Kern has received more than $17 million in grant funding from the Office of Special Education Programs, the National Institute of Mental Health, and a recent Center Grant from the Institute for Education Sciences. She is currently associate editor of both the *Journal of Behavioral Education* and *School Mental Health* and serves on the editorial boards of seven educational journals.